Heal
Arthritis

Heal
Arthritis

Physically—Mentally—Spiritually

The Edgar Cayce Approach

by William A. McGarey, M.D.

ASSOCIATION FOR
RESEARCH AND
ENLIGHTENMENT

A.R.E. Press • Virginia Beach • Virginia

A.R.E. Press

215 67th Street

Virginia Beach, VA 23451-2061

Note: All biblical quotations are taken from the New English Bible.

Library of Congress Cataloging-in-Publication Data
McGarey, William A.
Heal arthritis : physically—mentally—spiritually : the Edgar Cayce approach / William A. McGarey.
p.   cm.
ISBN 0-87604-399-6
ISBN 13: 978-0-87604-399-8
1. Arthritis—Alternative treatment. 2. Cayce, Edgar, 1877-1945. Edgar Cayce readings. I. Title.
RC933.M36   1998
616.7'2206—dc21   97-31083

Cover design by Kim Cohen and John Comerford

Contents

Foreword

Waiting in line at my neighborhood pharmacy recently, I was struck by the variety of arthritis painkillers on the counter next to the cash register. Aches and pains in the joints must be a pretty common complaint, I thought. The "deep penetrating power" of the creams and ointments promised quick relief for the buyer—and their prominent display no doubt delivered profitable sales for the druggist.

As it happened, I was reading the manuscript for this new book on arthritis at the time, and I was struck by the contrast. Whatever relief the pharmacist's remedies might bring would be temporary. *Heal Your Arthritis* by William A. McGarey, M.D., offers much more.

By the time I finished the book, I wished my mother

had lived long enough to hear Dr. McGarey's message. She suffered from nagging arthritis pains much of her adult life. She took cortisone tablets recommended by her physician. If they brought her momentary relief, it was clear that cortisone was no cure. A talented portrait painter, she was forced to give up her art in later years because it was too painful to hold a paintbrush. She accepted the doctor's advice that there was no known cure for arthritis. I feel sure if she had been a patient of Dr. McGarey's, she would not have been obliged to retire her paints and palette. For, as he describes its causes, arthritis results from "improper bodily functions" that can be reversed.

Indeed, the author declares that "the common denominator of causes of arthritis is lack of proper eliminations." He broadens our awareness of what this means by emphasizing the detoxifying work of the lymphatic system, which he notes is usually overlooked in this connection. The lymph glands "provide the very first step in accepting the waste products from the cells of the body, along with the other products that the cells create, and carry them to the thoracic duct, thence to the venous system, to travel through the lungs and the heart and thence to be eliminated through the liver and the intestines, kidneys, lungs or the skin."

His simple explanation of the lymph glands makes me realize how little we understand the most basic functions of our own bodies, and thus how much we take for granted and even how badly we neglect this wonderful mechanism, the body, that was not designed to be a house of pain. Not too long ago we published in *Venture Inward* magazine, for which Dr. McGarey is a distinguished health consultant, an article on a new therapy known as manual lymph drainage—one of the many new holistic treatments that are available to help those of us who are determined to help our bodies function properly.

When Dr. McGarey writes of bodily functions, however, he does so in the broadest sense to include not just the physical body but the mind and spirit as well, for all three play a vital part in creating good or ill health, including arthritis. Thus he tells us that a good diet, a positive attitude, and a faithful spirit will all go a lot further than the pharmacist's quick fixes in overcoming and preventing this painful affliction.

One has to admit that he offers no "magic bullets." And yet there is one magical remedy in his bag of alternative medicine: human energy. "The energy emitted by every human being can heal, can move objects, make plants grow," writes McGarey. "And we must always remember that the energy coming from us is always divine energy coming through us. We are the channels for that energy."

Human energy is a powerful healing force that he assures us is readily available, and without a prescription. We can all tap into it in order to gain and preserve good health, for it is the power of the Divine. Dr. McGarey is no old-fashioned "faith healer" but a New Age alternative-medicine practitioner who respects the power of this universal force because he has seen it work in the healing of his patients. His authority for explaining it in cosmological terms is Jesus of Nazareth. McGarey writes: "It's much like what Jesus told His disciples: 'It is the Father who dwells in me doing His own work.' [Edgar] Cayce elaborated on that statement in one of his readings, quoting Jesus: 'I of myself may do nothing, but as the Father workest in me, through me.' "

So, while my pharmacist touts pain relievers that are temporary at best, Dr. McGarey goes to the very root of this condition and offers guidance for permanent relief.

Overcoming arthritis is possible, he promises, if we are willing and able to give ourselves—body, mind, and spirit—the opportunity to be whole. That may require some radical lifestyle changes, such as giving up fast foods, fried foods especially; getting regular exercise instead of vegetating in front of the TV; and finding ways to minimize the stress in our lives, at home as well as on the job. Some of his proscription may require the supreme sacrifice, such as giving up "fussing with your spouse at mealtime."

In a word, we are challenged to take responsibility for whatever condition we are in if we wish to improve our health. And while that approach may not yield overnight results, they may be more lasting. Thus, even arthritis may be a blessing if it forces us to take a personal inventory of how we are living out our lives. If we respond positively to its challenge, the reward can be high indeed—not just deliverance from pain, but a more lasting sense of vibrant health.

A. Robert Smith
Editor
Venture Inward

Preface

Let's Go on a Spiritual Journey!

ↄ

Edgar Cayce, widely known as the best-documented psychic of the twentieth century, would, for many decades, lie down on a couch, close his eyes, clasp his hands across his abdomen, and relax into a state of altered consciousness. As the conductor of the readings gave him directions, he would correctly describe the illness—or the physiological abnormalities—of the subject, who might be a few feet or perhaps thousands of miles distant from where Cayce was giving the reading.*

*The Cayce readings are identified by a file number assigned to the person, group, or topic for whom the readings was given. The first set of numbers refers to the individual, while the second is the order given in that series. For example, 849-4 identifies the fourth reading given for the person assigned number 849.

Then he would make suggestions that, when followed, would help the person to recover even when many doctors had failed to be of significant help.

Until he died in 1945, Cayce gave nearly 15,000 such readings, two-thirds of them dealing with illness and healing. They were all unique and personal to the individual receiving the reading, reflecting Cayce's universal awareness that each person is, in reality, different from every other person in the earth. The readings were found to be remarkably accurate; they brought to the inquirer a wealth of information about our creation and destiny, our entry into the earth's environment again and again, and our experiences throughout many of those lifetimes. Reincarnation, for Cayce, became simply a fact. And he maintained that every experience is an opportunity for soul growth.

Cayce's readings have gained him the status of a seer to many who have studied his work, which is housed in the A.R.E. (Association for Research and Enlightenment, Inc.) library at 67th Street and Atlantic Avenue in Virginia Beach, Virginia. He is probably best known for his predictions of earth changes and the changes in our consciousness that would come about between the years 1958 and 1998. But for those who have worked in the Search for God study groups and designed their lives to manifest the Christ Consciousness as well as they could, Cayce's readings have left a life-changing legacy.

They proved to be life-changing for me. I first heard of the man in 1955, some ten years after he died. But his insights into our nature and our relationship to God led me to recognize and acknowledge the Creative Forces present and active in every person I meet, and in every patient I encounter in my practice of medicine. It altered my approach to my patients, moving me to treat them more effectively and naturally as a true union of body, mind, and spirit.

During the forty years I have worked with this material, I've incorporated the essence of it into the books I've written and in a similar manner into my life. I've seen thousands of individuals awaken to a deeper relationship with their fellow humans and with the Force we call God. In the process, many have found the riches behind the illnesses they have overcome in the spiritual journey they pursued because of these readings.

It is for these reasons and because of my own journey that I am dedicating this book to Edgar Cayce, with whom I must have had some past-life relationships in the practice of healing the body—perhaps in Persia or the Holy Land. Were it not so, I doubt I would have focused so deeply into the universal fund of knowledge contained in these readings. And, although he is no longer in the earth plane, I sincerely and deeply thank him.

William A. McGarey, M. D.
A.R.E. Clinic
Phoenix, Arizona

Introduction

༄

He becomes a physician when he speaks
of That which is unknown,
unmarked, and efficacious.

Paracelsus

In a 1990 study published by the Center for Disease Control, thirty-eight million people were reported to have one form or another of arthritis. Seven million were significantly impaired in their work, home, or daily activities. Other sources vary in their estimates.

Drug companies, doctors, and health-care providers make part of their income from those who suffer from arthritis. The patient and the family members, however, are all involved in trying to bring about—with the help of others—a resolution to the problem. Arthritis always brings with it pain and discomfort, frustration, a degree of depression or anger, with resentment directed toward either the body, the elements, the heredity, or whatever it may be that brought about the aching joints and disability. Most often the patient directs his anger outside, and those who apparently do not deserve those emotional experiences share with the patient the difficulties and hurts that come inevitably with painful, chronic illnesses. Arthritis, with all of its disturbances, difficulties, and misery, has continued to harass us over the centuries. So there is a question that must be asked.

Can Arthritis Really Be Healed?

I have no question in my mind that arthritis *can* be healed. Why would I, as a physician, bring psychic information into a discussion of a physical disease as widespread as arthritis if I did not believe wholeheartedly that this is the case? I have spent more than forty years studying and applying concepts of healing from Edgar Cayce's unconscious mind in my practice of medicine and found that they work! And they worked consistently.

But What About This "Spiritual Journey"?

Why would this information point out to any individual that he or she has embarked on something usually talked about only in the context of a religious experience—or a vision—not really found in an illness? For one thing, Cayce viewed every experience as an opportunity for soul growth. Moreover, his readings talked about consciousness of the cells, the organs, the glands and the systems of the functioning body—and even indicated the very atoms which make up all of the structures of the body have their own kind of consciousness. Arthritis is not simply a disease. It deals with the consciousness of the individual and explains to an extent the reason we are on a journey at all. For we are truly seeking a goal that lies some distance ahead of us, certainly, and it involves our becoming cocreators with the Source of all life, the Force we call God.

The material coming from the sleeping body of this man Cayce gave information on a wide variety of illnesses always helpful and sometimes totally effective in bringing about resolution of a disease. Healing comes about through establishing a harmony inside the body.

Living out in one's life, according to these readings, the fruits of the Spirit of Love does bring about soul growth, a more peaceful environment inside the body, and a coordination where the functions of the body can then create a more balanced state of health. This, in turn, allows an improvement in the aching bones. Living out the fruits of the Spirit flows over into the mind and the emotions, touching the spirit of the whole person, who reaps the benefit, the harmony that has been promised.

So it is that in an illness such as arthritis, we can find ourselves on a Spiritual Journey as we move toward overcoming the illness. But there are many more questions to ask. They are all valid. We need to look, in a sense, behind the illness rather than at the simple manifestation of it. You may ask me, for instance:

"What Can You Do to Cure Me of Arthritis?"

Of course, my obvious answer is I don't cure anyone of anything. I may give you a guide to go by to arrive at a certain place, but I do not take the trip for you. Healing is always a spiritual event within the cells and consciousness of the body itself, and you must make yourself willing to allow healing to come about. That's the part you play.

There is as much of the God-Force flowing through you as there was flowing through the body of Jesus two thousand years ago. The big difference is that He knew what love was; He manifested it completely and His body was filled with the divine force of life. He had no obstructions. You do. So do I.

How do we get over arthritis, then? Sometimes simple medicines can do the trick. Apparently. But they rarely correct the cause; if you stop the medication, the symptoms usually reappear. So we need to look beyond the symptoms at the cause of those abnormalities in the function of the physical body that seem to bring the "disease" into reality.

We need to talk about assimilation and elimination. We need to ask about the pH of the body tissues, the acid-alkaline balance throughout the body. We need to look at what we are eating. And, perhaps, why we are constipated, not eliminating properly. And we need to look at the thoughts and the emotions we are harboring within the deeper recesses of our minds. For they are indeed important in bringing about healing in the body or creating the disease that afflicts us.

What about our lifestyle—does it have any effect on how our body functions? What part does stress play in the cause or correction of arthritis. How much sleep do we get? What is our relationship with our family and friends, and those at work—harmonious? Frustrated? Do you smoke, for instance? How about exercise? What about prayer and meditation? Are these part of your routine? Have you been studying your dreams and the symbology dreams offer us? And, of course, what is arthritis, anyhow? How does it start? What parts of the body are affected? Does one's attitude have any part to play in the cause, course, or correction of arthritis?

We can say that healing comes about in any human body through reversal of those abnormalities that brought the illness into being. Can bones and joints and tendons and synovial sacs be returned to normal? If so, is that healing? These questions need to be explored, especially for the student of the body who is a true seeker of the truth. Can we see the body, for instance, as it really is—as a conglomeration of energies, atoms flying around at the speed of light or faster, creating structure out of mind, electricity, and function?

Why would we attempt to upgrade the immune system in treating arthritis? What is the benefit to be received from counseling in regard to emotions? How would a "balancing" of the functions of the seven major endocrine glands bring about an improvement in the joints or muscles of the body? Lots of questions, but all are pertinent to understanding the body and what might be done to bring about healing. The information from the Cayce material needs to be explored in reference to all these questions; it can supply a foundation for those who seek to overcome and reverse the process (condition) we call arthritis.

Cayce's picture of humankind explains, for us to understand our situation here on the earth, that we are possessed with eternal life, that we were in existence in a time predating the creation of the earth itself. All that has ever happened to us is contained within the memory bank that we carry around with us at all times. We are truly a visitor on this planet, a soul clothed in a three-dimensional body that can serve us well if we treat it right.

We need to think about ourselves as individuals who have the potential to overcome any illness that may affect us. We need to change our perspective—at least occasionally—to include these possibilities as virtual realities. We do have power that we have seldom, if ever, claimed as our own.

So let's start on our Spiritual Journey—even though we may call it arthritis!

1

How Does Healing Really Come About?
The Concepts

~

Millions of Americans suffer from arthritis and, with the help of their health-care providers, keep looking outside for a cause of the affliction, as if it must come from outside their bodies. "For why in the world would I ever inflict this kind of difficulty on me?" Yet it does come from within our own bodies, and if we pay close attention to the wisdom available to us—and has been available over the centuries—we can not only find the cause closer than we have ever imagined, but also stimulate those forces which too often lie dormant within to bring about what we can truly call a healing.

My medical training gave me some understanding of the physiology and anatomy of the human body, but my early years of study of the Bible created the spiritual hunger that was satisfied much later on when I discovered the Edgar Cayce psychic readings. For instance, Cayce said we are body, mind, and spirit. We had our origin as souls in a spiritual dimension before the earth was formed—we are truly ancient beings—and have come into this earth plane over and over again, seeking not only to learn necessary lessons here, but also seeking a path to lead us back to where we started, a oneness with the Creative Forces of the Universe, that power we call God.

To put this concept into a more visual form, we can see in the following illustration that we, as souls, were created as Spirit (S), the giver of life itself; Mind (M), always the builder; and Will (W), the power to choose. This took place in the spiritual dimension. It naturally follows that the Soul is spiritual in its very essence. When we come into the earth plane, we die to the spiritual environment and are born into the earth, through the medium of our mother's womb.

In the earth we, as souls, take on a three-dimensional form so that we can experience the earth environment. We become, then, Spirit, Mind, and Body. In the same illustration, the mind plays the part of the interlocutor between the spiritual and the physical, or body. The mind is the means of communication between our original soul-self and the physical body here in the earth.

Throughout our experiences since we were created, we have had the ability to choose, through the medium of the will. This is shown as a small triangle with a C in it. Our minds are constantly active, and thus use the power of the will, or the power to choose, in all of our relationships, even in choosing our parents. This is very important, because we then become responsible entities, making our lives what we wish. Our journey is marked by choices and formulated in that manner. During this

Created in the Image of God

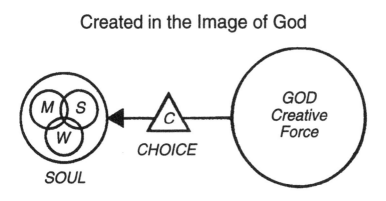

journey, consciousness, choices, and the powers in the uncharted depths of the unconscious mind bring our spiritual origin and our physical bodies closer together in what we call illness. We develop attitudes or emotions as we move along in our interpersonal relationships, and these—as habits lodged in the unconscious mind—alter the physiological functionings of our bodies through the powers invested in the hormonal and neurological activities of our endocrine glands. Most often these emotional habits are discounted in our unconscious minds as simply reactions. And we often excuse them by saying, "This is just the way I am." Very true, but "the way I am" is the way I have created myself to react. And the physiology bears the brunt of the reactions, whether they be positive or negative. Thus, we benefit or we end up hurting as a result of our responses, reactions, or our tendency to revert to a former state.

Edgar Cayce took the position, in his psychic readings, that there are no conditions of the human body which cannot be returned to normal. But he also insisted that conditions of illness, no matter what kind, have their origin in destructive activities which tend to lead the individual away from his or her chosen path back to God. This movement away from God became "sin" in the terminology of the readings. The healing of the illness was to aid in bringing about the adoption of a new awareness that might move a person once more back to the path and toward one's eventual, chosen goal Jesus, through a variety of methods—faith, touch, water and earth, prayer, the spoken word—healed all kinds of illnesses, physical, mental, and spiritual. These have been described by many as miraculous, although others say a miracle is a natural event that has not yet been understood. Of course, natural—in this use of the word—would then require that it be defined as encompassing not only the physical world, but also the spiritual and the mental. For we are body, mind, and spirit, and cannot be understood completely any other way.

It did not seem to matter to Jesus what was wrong with a person who came to Him for aid. In Mark 2:1-12, Jesus told a paralyzed man his sins were forgiven him. Then He told the scribes who were thinking "in their hearts" only God can forgive sins, "Why do you harbour thoughts like these? Is it easier to say to this paralyzed man, 'Your sins are forgiven,' or to say, 'Stand up, take your bed, and walk?' " Then He simply told the man to take up his bed and go on home, and the man did as he was told. It appears that Jesus saw illness as sin, and forgiveness such as he was able to offer (and describe) as the healing factor. Sometimes faith or touch brought about the same result of healing. In each instance there was, certainly, an awakening in consciousness—which can come about in any of us who truly believe Jesus was telling the truth.

Edgar Cayce gave suggestions for healing that sometimes included qualities of the Spirit, such as understanding and forgiveness; but also substances of the earth such as food, herbs, and oils, for instance. Any of these might bring relief to one who suffers from arthritis. He wove his comments around the concept that we are spiritual beings living in a three-dimensional world where we are presently visitors.

He repeatedly reminded us that the world and all it encompasses were brought into being by the same Creative Energies that created us. Things of the earth, then, all are manifestations of God and have their own specific abilities to bring healing to an ailing body.

Early in my experience with the Edgar Cayce readings, Fred showed up at the A.R.E. Clinic with a three-month history of swelling and redness in his right foot and ankle, as well as a recently developed back pain. His doctors had diagnosed him as having rheumatoid arthritis and his latex test for this condition was returned positive. Fred was sixty-five. Aside from these recent symptoms, he was in excellent health.

His therapy program followed very closely the suggestions given in the Cayce readings for working on this condition: Atomidine in series and in cycles, Epsom salts baths each week, full-body massages weekly, and then foot and ankle massages with peanut oil each night before retiring. He was also to use some visualization techniques, which we taught him, and follow certain dietary suggestions. His response was rapid. In two months, the swelling was gone, there was no discomfort and no stiffness, and, to all intents and purposes, he was well. Follow-up revealed his recovery promised to be permanent.

What Is Healing?

Since the day my activities became aligned with the Edgar Cayce information, I have repeatedly asked myself, "What is healing?" We need to ask that question. My training in medical school did not give me information to satisfy my questioning mind. The field of medicine is not a healing profession. The fields of chiropractic, osteopathy, naturopathy, physical therapy, acupuncture—these are not healing professions—not as they exist today. They are approaches toward correction of an illness and as such do an excellent job when used sensibly. However, that is not the same as healing.

Healing is always a process. It is not treating a diagnosed illness—healing is treating the living, ongoing functional unit we call the human body, with its mind, its spirit, and its emotions. All have shared in creating the problem, and thus must take part in the healing, and unless all factors are considered in starting the process of a return back to normal, there is no true healing—just, as Cayce put it, " . . . a healer for dollars and cents!" (2739-2) True healing can be accomplished only when the spiritual nature of the human being is recognized as divine; when the mind of the one in need is activated (either from within or without) to put into action concepts of healing in his/her own body; and when the body is treated in such a manner that physiological abnormalities are restored to normal. For healing to occur, a change in consciousness must come about; a new direction in life must be brought about—in other words, a divine happening must occur within the consciousness of the cells and atoms of the body itself.

To aid others in the healing process, we must truly look at our fellow human beings as having been created by God, in His image; with a mind that is the builder; and a body, the result of the mind being active and creative, using the Spirit as the force of creation itself. This is the story given in the Edgar Cayce material, which has been available for the better part of a century.

Physical healing can often be observed by others; when one who has arthritis can move one's fingers freely—this can be seen by others. But what about the feelings, the disturbing emotions, the fears the person experiences—which often lead to illnesses of the physical or a recurrence of the illness if they are not eliminated? Are these to be relieved instantly, or is this healing also a process? Can they be observed easily from outside, or do they remain hidden to the casual observer? I received a letter from an artist who took part in one of our residential Temple Beautiful Programs. She was grateful to all those who helped her and made that experience the "most important eleven days of my life!"

She wrote: "I arrived confused, frightened, expectant—yet doubtful. I was exhausted from trying to make sense of all my thoughts and feelings: What are these terrible pains in my body? Why am I on the verge of tears much of the time? What is this feeling that if I can just see over the next mountain, I will know where to go? But, which path? How far? Can I make it alone? I learned the answer: I needed the love and support, wisdom and guidance of others to help me find and follow my path to healing my body, mind, and spirit. I am stronger now for being able to ask for help.

"I learned that the pain in my body was caused by a combination of physical, emotional, and spiritual issues which I have now addressed on all levels. Now I am free from pain most of the time. When it recurs even for a moment, I know my body is signaling me to pay attention. It is a guide instead of an enemy. I feel joyous most of the time. My tears are now mostly from feeling touched by love, beauty, or from missing the wonderful family of friends I made during those eleven magic days at the Oak House.

"I now feel free to be the powerful, beautiful, loving person that I am, but was afraid to be. The lesson learned is that we are all powerful, beautiful, and loving for we

are made in God's image. You have given me the gift of
new life. I know now that my path is to spread love and
light in all that I do."

So, eleven days—or in Fred's case, two months—it is
always a process, this healing of human ills. And the soul
growth that ensues enlightens the world in its own way.
One of the principles of healing which comes from the
Cayce readings gives us food for thought:

. . . all *healing* is from the Divine within, and not
from medications. Medications only *attune* or accord a body for the proper reactions from the el-
emental forces of divinity within each corpuscle,
each cell, each muscle, each activity of every atom
of the body itself. 1173-6

. . . no medicine, no mechanical appliance *does*
the healing. It only attunes the body to a perfect
coordination and the Divine gives the healing.

For Life is divine, and each atom in a body that
becomes cut off by disease, distrust or an injury,
then only needs awakening to its necessity of coordination, cooperation with the other portions that
are divine, to *fulfill* the purpose for which the body,
the soul, came into being. 1173-7

This offers a different perspective, doesn't it? We always have the opportunity to look at things differently,
and it is part of an awakening process. Then, healing
one's body might indeed come about. If not total healing, at least a step in that direction. For the internal se-
creting glands and the body's physiology will start the
healing process. Open-mindedness is the first step in
acquiring not only the understanding needed, but the
wisdom from applying that understanding. What does

all this mean to us today? My analysis is that we have the essence of how healing comes about right here in our grasp, those of us who have accepted, studied, and applied in our lives these concepts of healing, no matter where we learned them.

Castor Oil Packs

Although Velma had no problem with arthritis, her experiences provide another example of how a simple application can restore order in the body physiology. Velma had a hysterectomy in 1965. The surgery went along all right, it seemed, but for twenty-three years she experienced constant gaseous distention, constipation, abdominal miseries, edema of the ankles, and episodes where her "gut" would feel as if it were twisting on itself. These periods lasted sometimes for hours. After being seen as a patient at the clinic, she was instructed on how to use a castor oil pack. She was faithful in following instructions and came back for a recheck in two weeks.

She told us that after the very first pack was placed on her abdomen, within minutes she felt as if the gut inside her belly wall untwisted on itself—and since that time there had been no recurrence of symptoms, no twisting sensations. Her ankles were no longer edematous, her abdominal "miseries," constipation, and gaseous distention were all gone.

Healing comes in many disguises. I've seen it happen all at once. Some would call this a miracle, but when one considers that the body, the mind, and the spirit are all one, then it begins to look more like we have touched the true nature of the body as God brought it into being. We are indeed composed of energy in the form of atoms, and all energy is a manifestation of the Creative Force we call God. To touch the body that is ill at times brings

healing. Jesus knew this, and even those who touched
His robe sometimes experienced body healing—or was
it healing of the Spirit? Or perhaps the mind? Why should
it be one and not all three? All of these things are mysteries of the world we live in, a world created in the first
place as a workshop in which we could find our way back
to the Force that first brought us into being. So we are
indeed surrounded by mysteries, aren't we?

In my experience with healing and with the Cayce readings, castor oil with its healing qualities has probably
brought me the greatest rewards while providing the
most in the way of laughter, fun, and joy. God must have
a tremendous sense of humor to endow something so
common and disregarded by the most of humankind with
a vibration that frequently brings health out of illness.
Literally thousands now have received healing of one
sort or another through the use of castor oil packs. And a
large percentage of those people have written us at the
Clinic, telling of their successes. When one uses this un-
usual oil on the surface of the skin, strange things happen inside the body. We keep on trying to explain the why
of the matter, but it still remains somewhat of a mystery.

In the late '80s, we received a research grant to study
some energy effects as they were described in the Cayce
readings. We chose the castor oil packs, since our experience in the A.R.E. Clinic with this approach to healing
had been used most extensively. Our pilot study was very
promising, but our funding source dried up before we
could go to step two. The conclusion we drew from the
work we did, however, led us to understand that a castor
oil pack placed over the liver area and upper right abdomen for one hour, in just one application, improved the
function of the immune system. We were excited, because our clinical work with thousands of patients gave
us the same conclusion.

It is only reasonable, in my mind, to understand the immune system—which has the duty of protecting the body from all kinds of difficulties and helps rebuild the body under all circumstances—can be benefited by the use of castor oil packs as a basic therapy for most any condition of illness in the human body. We followed this hypothesis for nearly three decades before we did the research, and we find it still works for those who use the packs. One of my recent books, *The Oil That Heals*, deals extensively with the use of these packs (see Appendix).

A young lady broke her jaw in an automobile accident. It was a multiple fracture, and the jaw had to be wired shut until it healed. The jaw was healing all right, but she had difficulty cleaning her teeth during the weeks she wore the braces. She told me, "All my food was liquefied, but there were small particles that stuck to the braces. It was becoming very uncomfortable and I was concerned about cavities and gum erosion. I was new in A.R.E. and had read about all the benefits of castor oil. I decided to try brushing my teeth with a drop or two of castor oil on my toothbrush. The effect was all I could have hoped for. My teeth felt clean and the soreness from the wires disappeared. The end result was no cavities and minimal gum erosion. I still use it often and I have very good teeth."

It has always seemed to me that healing takes time, in the same manner the development of an illness takes time. This realization led me to understand the physiological processes of the body were the only life supports of the body and they keep on acting either beneficially or destructively through the passage of time. Thus we become ill or achieve health through the activity we call time.

If castor oil does indeed reduce inflammation, then the body was able to heal the gums despite the irritation from the wires. The tissues of the mouth were able to eliminate irritating substances more easily because of the oil, and the total effect was healing of tissues, no cavities, minimal gum erosion during those weeks, and the feeling of health and cleanliness in the mouth. In other words, health. Thousands of individuals over the years have told me of their personal experiences with castor oil, great and small, over one form of illness or another. We could say healing comes about through stimulating the liver or relieving pain, reducing toxemia or increasing lymphatic circulation, etc. But it doesn't tell us the answer to the question: "How does castor oil heal?"

Castor oil is usually placed on the outside of the body. In order to reach the liver, for instance, it would have to penetrate through the tissues to the liver in a vibratory manner and create a biochemical effect on the liver internally. Or perhaps an electromagnetic result might show us the answer. Evidence in the future will help.

Every story that comes to me in the mail is different. Sometimes the manner in which healing comes about is totally another mystery. Dianne told me how she had injured her heel and plantar arch of her foot while exercising. The condition was diagnosed as fasciitis, an inflammation and possible infection of a tendon torn in that area of the foot. She was nearly immobilized from the pain, especially while walking.

She first saw her chiropractor, who worked on her lower lumbar area. It did not help. Then she had acupuncture treatments, which helped only temporarily. Next she got arch supports from her family doctor, which did not bring relief. Finally, she saw an orthopedic doctor who supplied the correct diagnosis and gave her an anti-inflammatory drug.

"After two months," she said, "there was fifty percent improvement, but after four months, the condition still was not cleared up. Still painful to walk. So I got out my castor oil at 2:00 a.m. one morning—maybe a dream-inspired event—and I made a poultice of cotton soaked in the oil, covered with plastic, and wrapped up in an elastic bandage, and went to bed again. It worked. At least there was a tingling vibration in the foot from the arch to the heel. Then, for a week, I applied the pack at night, then discontinued for two days. Then on again for three more days. On the eleventh night, when I put the pack on, I noticed a large blister about the size of a half dollar, 1/8th of an inch thick, and located on the inside of my heel, just below my ankle."

When she wrote the letter, the pain had decreased markedly. Several months later, she wrote that "the blister which appeared on my heel was carried away by the bloodstream within a month. Neither the pain nor swelling has ever returned. My foot has been perfect ever since."

Healing the Body Touches the Divine

We seldom relate true healing to our spiritual adventure here on the Earth. We usually want to achieve a better state of health so we can go about doing what we have planned to do. But there is a relationship between healing and the Divine, and we can describe it in many ways. Let's agree that we are originally spiritual beings. Our spiritual body—different from but part of the physical body—is a vibratory unit, in some manner attuned to the Creative Forces of the Universe from which we derive our life and our being.

Healing, then, in order to affect the vibratory unit, must be vibratory in nature. Everything in this dimension is, in one manner or another, vibratory. All things are composed of atoms, which are in constant motion.

So all things are in essence vibratory.

Some substances, however, in their vibratory form, are destructive when applied to the human body, while others are very helpful, very constructive. All substances emit vibrations, so, as part of their nature, are either constructive or destructive.

An article published in the Austin *American Statesman* (Dec. 11, 1988) shows the castor bean in a new light. From the castor bean comes castor oil. Also, the plant, the *Ricinus communis*, produces in the bean a substance called ricin, which is both poisonous and healing. Ricin has been used to cure leukemia in laboratory animals, but the bean, containing the ricin, can be poisonous to humans if ingested. Researchers at the University of Texas Southwestern Medical Center in Dallas have used ricin to kill the HIV virus that causes AIDS. The ricin is released into a laboratory solution containing cells infected by HIV. In the study, it was found the ricin seeks out the virus and the virus-infected cells and kills them. Other research has linked ricin to another substance that will penetrate cells infected with the AIDS virus, thus allowing the ricin to destroy the virus inside the cell.

No one has yet postulated how the activity comes about vibrationally, but it has been suggested the biochemical action interferes with the life of the virus. Yet biochemical activity is always electrical, or vibrational.

When the oil from the castor bean is applied to the skin of an individual, strange things happen, which are very difficult to explain. A friend of mine from Wisconsin fractured one of the small bones of her foot, which did not heal. She wanted to resume jogging, but the pain was too great. Then a light went on in her head, in a sense, and she thought, "I'll try castor oil." She applied a small pack to her foot regularly, and the pain started to go away. Now she just rubs some castor oil into the back of her foot and any pain present disappears. And she has resumed jogging. She also found that the same kind of pack applied to a thrombosed hemorrhoid would bring rapid relief and healing for her.

Peanut Oil

Oils bring about different responses when applied to the body. Perhaps this is a vibrational response also. Why did Cayce, for instance, suggest castor oil packs for liver problems, and peanut oil massages for arthritic joints? Another of my correspondents found her left ankle was stiffening up and becoming painful, with the pain starting to migrate up her leg. She knew about castor oil and so applied it with an overlying bandage. But it did no good. She prayed, and "like lightening" the answer came to her to use peanut oil. She did, and the pain and stiffness disappeared at once! It's difficult for me to realize sometimes how rapidly healing can occur, but with this lady it took five minutes. Was her spiritual body directly affected? We don't really know. But don't try to tell this woman it didn't happen!

Human Energy

The energy emitted by every human being can heal, can move objects, make plants grow or wither away—it indeed has many facets. What is the energy? It has vibrational qualities—not yet fully understood—but is also electrical in its nature. Cayce indicated all energies are vibrational in nature. When you place your hands on another person, there is the movement of that energy, either to help or to hinder although this is not necessarily a conscious choice. The changes that occur within the body reflect the desire, the direction, the ideals of the one who does the touching. And we must always remember that the energy coming *from* us is always divine energy coming *through* us. We are the channels for that energy.

It's much like what Jesus told His disciples: "It is the Father who dwells in me doing his own work." (John: 14:10) Cayce elaborated on this statement in one of his readings, quoting Jesus: "I of myself may do nothing, but as the Father worketh in me, through me." Then, in the same reading (1299-1) Cayce said, "Know then that the force in nature that is called electrical or electricity is that same force ye worship as Creative or God in action!" It gives us much to think of, for the same electrical force that allows us as individuals to move and speak and breathe is that same force that moved through Jesus and which allowed Edgar Cayce to give readings.

Healing in the human body, whether it comes from a manipulation (chiropractic, osteopathic); from touching (massage, healing touch, prayer—these are all related); from the use of castor oil or a substance related to that oil; from peanut oil; or from the vibration set up within the body when placed in an electromagnetic field or treated with electrotherapy; healing comes about when the consciousness of the forces, the cells within the body come to the awareness of the Divine, that which brought all of us and all of these forces into being.

Remember, in healing we are influencing others, or being influenced by others, to create a greater unity between individuals and the God that created both them and the earth. This is what happens when you heal your own body or aid another in the healing process. Cayce said it like this:

For, all healing comes from the one source. And whether there is the application of foods, exercise, medicine, or even the knife—it is to bring [to] the consciousness of the forces within the body that aid in reproducing themselves—[which is] the awareness of creative or God forces. 2696-1

. . . all healing of every nature is the changing of the vibrations from within—the attuning of the Divine within the living tissue of a body to Creative Energies. This alone is healing. Whether it is accomplished by the use of drugs, the knife or whatnot, it is the attuning of the atomic structure of the living cellular force to its spiritual heritage. 1967-1

When I first began studying the Cayce material on healing, I learned that all healing comes from within; each healing experience (true healing, that is) is an adventure in soul growth and a step toward our eventual destiny of being one with God.

I remember my first experience as a channel of healing for someone else—not realizing what I'd done until it was all over. A young woman with multiple sclerosis, who was attending one of our Temple Beautiful Programs, was sitting in the front passenger seat of the car, when we brought her wheelchair around so that she could get out and go inside to the meeting. She turned around and grasped the door frame between the front and the back door with her right hand at the same time the man who was getting out from the back seat slammed the door shut without noticing her hand in the way. The door smashed her fingers. We quickly opened the door again.

We lifted her into her wheelchair and I instinctively took her hand and stood there holding it clasped between my two hands. I just wanted her to stop hurting. Gradually she quieted down and the pain, which had

brought tears to her eyes, went away. It took fifteen minutes, but when I wheeled her into the building, she
joined the rest of the group and had no more pain, no
swelling, and it was as if nothing had happened.
Was it the vibrations coming from my hands? Was it a
power, an energy—call it what you will? It seemed to me
her need and my willingness to act, along with her belief
something good could happen, allowed the power of the
Divine to move through me and her pain disappeared.
No swelling. Her M.S., however, was unchanged. That
sort of thing has not happened so dramatically in my
experience since, but I know that pain, swelling, arthritis, all sorts of disabilities, can be returned to a normal
state if one who desires enough becomes a channel of
healing. But we must move ourselves—our own selfish
wishes and desires—out of the way so healing can move
through us. There was a Cayce reading given that dealt
with healing and vibration:

> . . . as to how the garments worn by the Child
> [Jesus] would heal children. For the body being per-
> fect radiated that which was health, life itself. Just
> as today, individuals may radiate, by their spiritual
> selves, health, life, that vibration which is destruc-
> tive to dis-ease in any form in bodies. 1010-17

Healing of the human body, then, is dealt with in
many ways in the Cayce readings. Following is another
explanation that speaks directly to each of us as we move
along on our spiritual journey:

> For in each physical body (and with this body,
> [257]), there are the abilities for the body to revive,
> resuscitate, reorganize itself continuously. It is only
> the consciousness that the activities of the body

waste with age, care, fear, doubt or the like, that produces what ye term old age or decrepitness in the activities of the body physically and mentally. 257-191

My experience, as well as my knowledge of the Cayce readings, leads me to understand the very first item that should be tended to is one's spiritual path and relationship to the Divine. Very simply, Jesus said, "Seek ye first the Kingdom of God, and his righteousness, and all these things shall be added unto you." (Matt. 6:33) We are spiritual beings, traveling our path toward Oneness in this earthly domain. Thus we need to remind ourselves that our Origin and our Destiny lie in another dimension—we are indeed eternal beings. We are guests here, with opportunities always to learn how to Love one another. And ourselves.

Once that firm foothold is established, we need to use our own creativity in seeking out all those means available to *aid* us in the healing process that has begun inside our body, our mind, and our spirit. For it doesn't matter whether it is castor oil packs, a proper diet, lifestyle changes, or even the knife. But we need to believe it can happen, and thus become active and live the experience.

Then healing may come.

2

What's the First Step in Healing Arthritis? Begin! Do Something!

⤻

Some time ago, I reevaluated a patient in the Clinic who had been through the Temple Beautiful Program more than five years earlier. He looked a bit older and as though he had been through a lot of life's experiences. He was in his fifties and he unfolded for me how the last five years had been more eventful and stressful than any similar period in his entire life.

"His" arthritis was still disabling him, and instead of being less of a problem, it was obviously a greater burden. This, in spite of having had the experience of the Temple Beautiful Program and a therapy plan to follow when he returned home. So I inquired further. Why did he not improve in spite of the problems he was facing? It should be added here that he still "owned" the arthritis.

He couldn't let it go, couldn't (or wouldn't) claim the heritage for himself which says he was created in God's image and could act in that manner.

His diet had suffered the worst. The castor oil packs were only occasionally used. He took his Atomidine for two weeks and then forgot to take it, except once in a while. He could not take the Epsom salts hot baths because it was difficult to get into his small bathtub. His massages were sporadic; and the violet ray treatments he was supposed to be getting were virtually nonexistent. Besides, he worried constantly because of the problems he still had resulting from his divorce about six years prior to his first visit to the Clinic.

He sheepishly admitted he had not been consistent with his therapy; he did not persist—and he certainly was not patient with his body and the way it responded. This state of affairs reminded me of one of Edgar Cayce's remarks about these qualities:

> Do as we have given, and we will bring the near normal conditions for this body. Be persistent, but be *consistent* with the applications—also, don't expect the results in one treatment! For it's been many seasons coming on! 5503-1

It's obvious to one who suffers from back pain that the effort to bring his physical body back to normal after he has developed what we call arthritis is met most often with at least a degree of failure. Sometimes no success at all. Any practicing physician knows the results of any therapeutic program can be negated by the recipient if he or she doesn't really believe something good is going to happen.

It's important, then, to start off this spiritual journey with success. On the baseball field, it is disheartening to come to bat in the last half of the first inning after our opponent (like the negative aspects of our unconscious minds) has put us ten runs behind.

Let's not do it that way. We want to take one step toward the goal and make it a roaring success. Then we can take another, and another, and so on. But let's be patient. Let's love our body sufficiently to be consistent in working with it. And let's persist!

In the story I just told, George admitted his diet had suffered the worst. It may be that following a good diet was the most difficult goal for him to attain. Nevertheless, diet is perhaps the very first step we need to take to restore an ailing body back to a state of health. Let's at least work on that hypothesis.

The rest of the steps might best be taken after we establish our success with diet. In the next few chapters, we can consider how our body really works and what and who we truly are. We would then be better equipped to continue our journey.

Let's look then at the concepts found for the most part in the Edgar Cayce readings, directed at people who have arthritis.

Arthritis Diet—Basic Principles

1. Eat liberal amounts of fruits and vegetables—fresh if possible, frozen or dried second best. Include a large raw vegetable salad as one main meal daily. Combine raw vegetables with gelatin often.

Plenty of lettuce should always be eaten by most *every* body; for this supplies an effluvium in the bloodstream itself that is a destructive force to *most* of those influences that attack the bloodstream. It's a purifier. 404-6

2. Watch acid-alkaline balance.
3. Avoid certain food combinations.
4. Balance foods grown above and below the ground, three above to one below. Eat more leafy vegetables than pod-type.

Although Cayce died in early 1945, his suggestions about what foods are best are basically those which the American Heart Association and others are now recommending. Health food stores abound today in our country, and most supermarkets make available for the consumer a wide variety of fresh fruits and vegetables, although they have as much salted fried potato chips and soft drinks as they do some of the better food choices one might make.

Fats are avoided by those who are seeking to have a healthier body while losing weight. The acid/alkaline balance in the body will be discussed later on in this book. But it is not difficult to remember that fruits and vegetables are nearly all alkaline reacting, while sweets, starches, and proteins are acid reacting. In planning your diet, take four alkaline foods to one that produces acid ash. These can be distributed throughout the three daily meals to make sense in your planning. Cayce stimulates our thinking in many ways. In the following excerpt, he talks about a rule and then reminds us, in a sense, that we sometimes must make our own rules about our diet:

> ... have rather a percentage of eighty percent alkaline-producing to twenty percent acid-producing foods. Then, it is well that the body not become as one that couldn't do this, that or the other; or as a slave to an idea of a set diet. Do not take citrus fruit juices *and* cereals at the same meal. Do not take milk or cream in coffee or in tea. Do not eat fried

foods of any kind. 1568-2

While you are taking steps to reverse the process in
your body that caused you to develop arthritis, please be
aware that peace, not warfare, produces healing. Cayce
said that never "under strain, when very tired, very excited, very mad, should the body take foods in the system . . . And never take any food that the body finds is
not agreeing with same . . . " (137-30) In my experience,
these conditions—including fussing with your spouse at
mealtime—bring about an acid condition in the tissues
of the body and make things worse for anyone trying to
rebuild health in the body.

Certain food combinations that should be avoided
will be listed for your use later on in this chapter. One of
the principles listed above—foods grown above or below the ground—may still have some mystery associated
with it. I don't think it has to do with the chemicals involved, although they may play a part in the chemical
reactions of the body. But potatoes, beets, radishes, carrots, etc., are the "earthy" kind of food. Carrot tops, beet
tops, lettuce, etc., on the other hand, develop their values in the air and have a "light" kind of effect. The difference may be that the former are more starchy and tend
to produce an acid ash more so than the latter. Until the
full story comes out, and we do not know when that will
be—it's a good rule to follow.

Cayce added two footnotes to the use of vegetables in
the diet:

Include in the diet often raw vegetables prepared
in various ways, not merely as a salad but scraped
or grated and combined with gelatin . . . 3445-1

Q. Please explain the vitamin content of gelatin . . .

A. It isn't the vitamin content but it is [its] ability to work with the activities of the glands, causing the glands to take from that absorbed or digested the vitamins that would not be active if there is not sufficient gelatin in the body. 849-75

If part of your habit pattern is to grab a hamburger and a large order of french fries, think again. It does not help. Rather, it hinders your search for healing. So, read on.

Do Not Eat

1. White, bleached, or refined flour or grains or products made from these processed foods.
2. Refined sugar, raw sugar, brown sugar, molasses, or products made with these—such as jams, marmalades, ice cream, pastries, or candies.
3. Chocolate.
4. Milk or cream (very small amounts of milk allowed).
5. Pork (including bacon), beef, or veal.
6. Fat, especially animal fat.
7. Fried foods.
8. Canned (tinned) foods.
9. Spices or highly seasoned food.
10. Alcohol.
11. Beer, malt drinks, or carbonated water (soft drinks).
12. Starchy foods.
13. Cabbages, apples, bananas, strawberries, or fresh tomatoes.

Most of these selections can be easily recognized as being valid. Most of them taste good but, in one sense, are bitter to the belly. In other words, you might choose to look at them from a different perspective. Look at what might be good when it gets acted on by your digestive juices. That would then be constructive and healing. Whole wheat bread, for instance; avoiding those sweet and chocolate things; cutting way down on the milk. You'll find lots of fat in most protein servings, so you can rule those out, along with alcohol and soft drinks. Starchy foods are not so good to rebuild with.

But how did cabbage, apples, bananas, strawberries, and fresh tomatoes get on this list? Let's explore some of the readings.

I've included comments from three readings that seem to tell the story about tomatoes. Two were given to an individual with arthritis, one was not—this one given for a fifty-seven-year-old man who had diabetic tendencies and was eating a lot of tomatoes at the time:

Quite a dissertation might be given as to the effect of tomatoes upon the human system. Of all the vegetables, tomatoes carry most of the vitamins in a well balanced assimilative manner for the activities in the system. Yet if these are not cared for properly, they may become very destructive to a physical organism; that is, if they ripen after being pulled, or if there is the contamination with other influences.

In *this* particular body, as we find, the reactions from these have been not *always* the *best*. Neither has there been the normal reaction from the eating of same. For it tends to make for an irritation or humor. Nominally, though, these should form at least a portion of a meal three or four days out of every week; and they will be found to be *most* helpful.

The tomato is one vegetable that in most instances (because of the greater uniform activity) is preferable to be eaten after being canned, for it is then much more uniform.

The reaction in this body, then, has been to form
an acid of its own; though the tomato is among
those foods that may be taken as the *non*-acid
forming. But these should be of the best in *every* instance where they are used. 584-5

Cayce said in a number of instances that tomatoes
should be used only when picked ripe off the vine. The
next two selections were given in cases of arthritis and
expand on the use of tomatoes or their avoidance:

The diet will be those as have been outlined, ab-
staining from meats or butter, but as much of the
vegetable forces as possible; especially tomatoes—
these are *well* for the body, *properly* prepared. The
fruit only when well ripened on the vine; not as
gathered green and ripened afterward. That that is
well ripened, seasoned with salt, pepper, and if vinegar is preferable—or sugar and vinegar—this
would be well to use with same. 849-4

Noons—only raw green vegetables, as tomatoes
(this doesn't sound like much for this type, yet it
would be well if not too much is taken; one slice or
one quarter will not be too much, provided it is cut
well with), lettuce, *green* cabbage, celery, carrots,
spinach, onions, radish, and the like. These *green,
fresh, crisp;* never any of the wilted or withered, but
use more *outside* leaves than inside of the vegetables or the salad leaves or the like. Such a salad
may be taken with either oil or mayonnaise dressing. 932-1

We have used for some of our patients a three-day
apple diet, where only apples—the jenneting type (such

as so-called delicious apples)—are used as food for three days. Cayce called it a cleansing or detoxifying diet. But he had more to say about apples.

Baked apples are best in most instances, but there always are exceptions, undoubtedly because each human being has a unique set of physiological organs and systems. When there is anxiety or stress, raw apples are definitely contraindicated, as are fruits which are acid-producing. Baked apples certainly supply certain vitamins, but, as Cayce often said, "Beware of apples in any form, unless *well* cooked." This advice was for a young lady of twenty-eight years (2261-1) who had trouble with eliminations. It is important to remind you here that arthritis is basically a disease of faulty eliminations.

In Cayce's unconscious mind, both apples and bananas add silicon to the system when taken in certain ways. He apparently was convinced, in his psychic awareness, that silicon is definitely harmful for the body in certain instances or combinations. Apples baked, no problem. Bananas, he said, to beware of these, too. He explained this more definitively to a sixty-five-year-old woman who was in poor health generally.

> Do not overtax the system with bananas, unless these are ripened in their natural state; for the activity of these in the beginnings of their deterioration—before they are palatable—makes for a hardship upon the system. But those that are overripe, or that have been gathered or prepared when they have fully matured, may be taken in moderation at certain meals or times. 658-15

Cayce saw bananas, then, as being very helpful for individuals who are debilitated for one reason or another. But not usually for the arthritic person.

Strawberries seem to be in the same category—well to be taken in some instances, avoided in others. If one who has arthritis eats strawberries, they are best taken when in season and from one's own environment. And taken, too, in great moderation.

Cayce answered one woman's questions about her arthritis this way:

Q. May I eat strawberries . . . ?

A. These should be [taken] very little, not large quantities of these. A little would be very well, but not very much—and these occasionally . . .

Q. Any more advice regarding my diet?

A. As indicated, do not have those combinations that produce great acid. Citrus fruits while acid are *not* acid-producing, unless taken with quantities of starch. 1512-2

In my study of the Cayce suggestions about diet and nutrition, I have found each individual needs to remember that he or she is unparalleled in nature—all are worlds unto themselves. Each person is different in how their pylorus or appendix works as surely as their nose or their ears are different, or the way they walk. Thus the more reason one needs to look within always for the very best guidance as to diet and what needs to be taken or avoided.

But let's see what might be suggested as what foods would be good and helpful to include in your diet there at home and also when you are eating out at a restaurant or hotel.

These Foods Should Be Included in Your Diet

1. All kinds of raw vegetables (except cabbage): es-

pecially watercress, chard, mustard greens, kale, celery, carrots, lettuce (leaf or romaine).

2. Use only whole grain products. Black bread in moderation (pumpernickel, rye, or whole wheat).

3. Nuts, especially almonds and filberts. (Raw nuts are better than those roasted and salted).

4. Fish and seafood, fowl, lamb, wild game, liver, tripe, and pig knuckles (the only exception to no pork).

5. Vegetable juices, citrus fruit juices at times when cereal is not eaten.

6. Berries (see "strawberries" in previous list of foods to avoid) and citrus fruits.

7. Cooked leafy vegetables (except cabbage), pieplant (salsify), parsnips.

8. Potato peelings from the baked potato but not the bulk of it.

9. Jerusalem artichoke once each week.

10. A great deal of watercress and beet tops. (These especially help the eliminations.)

11. All fruits, preferably fresh, except apples, bananas, and strawberries (see previous list of foods to avoid).

12. Sweet milk and buttermilk in small amounts occasionally.

13. Small amounts of honey.

14. Use a vegetable seed oil or peanut/olive oil and vinegar salad dressing.

15. Small amounts of black coffee or tea.

16. Small amounts of cheese and two or three soft-cooked or poached eggs per week.

In the above list, cabbage is mentioned in items one and seven as foods not to be used. This needs a little explanation, for cabbage is indeed a great food. We need to remember that in osteoarthritis, there is an overacidity in the system. Frequently the acidity is brought on by too little sleep, work situations, arguments and disagreements, which create what we call stress. Often the stress is a constant companion.

Cayce pointed out in the following reading why cabbage needs special attention in the diet:

> When the body is under stress or strain by being tired, overactive, and then would eat heavy foods— as cabbage boiled with meat—these would produce acidity; yet cabbage *without* the meats would produce an alkaline reaction *under* the same conditions! 1411-2

Cayce emphasized this point in another reading given for a forty-five-year-old man with arthritis, while indicating how cabbage would still be a good food to eat.

> Eat plenty of . . . cabbage, all leafy vegetables, but not cooked in or with meat. Rather cook the vegetables in plain water, with a little butter or seasoning put on after being cooked, see? . . .
> Be mindful of the diet for a *long* period—at least six months to a year to two years; and the body will improve and keep better through the period. 2816-1

It should be noted cabbage is a good source of calcium, another reason why it should be treated with respect, especially in how it is prepared. It is always good, likewise, to cook cabbage by itself in Patapar or parchment paper, which retains the salts from the vegetable in the paper and can then be used as food instead of being thrown away.

Beet juice was recommended in the readings for arthritis, as well as for a number of other conditions. These two extracts partly explain the use of beet juice in the body:

Drink plenty of beet juice. Prepare this preferably
by cooking the beets in Patapar paper, so that all the
salts and juices that come from the beets may be
taken; about two ounces of this juice each day. 3672-1

The woman for whom the following reading was given
had arthritis associated with circulatory problems and
difficulty with assimilation and elimination:

In this body there should be taken, at least three
times each week, at least half an ounce to an ounce
of pure beet juice. This may include the leaves also.
Possibly it may be preferable from the cooked beets,
by themselves. But the beet juice should be ex-
tracted, or prepared as in a juicer; or, if this is not
practical for the body, then drink the juice in which
the beets are prepared—the water in which they are
boiled. But the pure juice is needed, not only the
salts but those elements that are within; which will
tend to alleviate these pressures and tendencies.
2946-1

People have asked me whether borscht (soup prepared from beets) would be good for the body in the case
of arthritis. I did not find borscht mentioned in the readings, but according to this bit of Cayce material, it seems
the soup would be good.

Next, let us look at some of the food combinations that
might be detrimental to the body in our search to overcome arthritis.

Avoid These Food Combinations

1. Starches and sweets at the same meal—too much
acidity.

2. Several starchy foods together—too much acidity.

3. Meat and potatoes—or meat and bread—or meat and starch together, upsets digestion.

4. Citrus fruits and cereals at the same meal—creates drosses in the body.

5. Coffee or tea with milk or cream—hard on digestion.

Through the abnormal functioning of the body, allergies are developed as well as distastes and inabilities to deal well with certain foods or certain combinations. There are undoubtedly many more combinations for some readers than are shown above.

With the guidelines and suggestions given in this chapter, you, as a traveler on your spiritual journey through the wastelands of arthritis, can begin to make specific steps toward healing through your diet. There are other steps to take, but this will get you started. It does not take perfection—it simply takes choices to improve here and there—and once you get started, you will feel the benefits in your body. So keep it up. But there's lots more to come.

3

How Do We Understand Arthritis—
The Energies Involved?

⌐

In understanding arthritis with the aid of medical textbooks, we can say nearly all cases of arthritis fall into one of two general classifications which are relatively easily differentiated, although poorly understood.

Atrophic arthritis, more commonly called rheumatoid, has also been given the name of proliferative arthritis or arthritis deformans. This type of disease process is characterized by inflammatory changes in the synovial membranes of the joints, in the structures surrounding the joints, and by a wasting away and decreasing density of the bones because of the absorption of mineral substances.

In the early stages there is a swelling that migrates from one joint to another; and stiffness of the joints occurs with a rather typical fusiform swelling of the inter-phalangeal joints (of the fingers) closest to the hands. Later on there is a malformation and fixation of the joints, and frequently an ulnar deviation of the fingers as a sign of this disease. Subcutaneous nodules are frequent and usually the disease is found beginning in young people, more commonly the male than the female.

The patient experiences anemia, chronic weight loss, loss of calcium in the bone structures, and is often rather severely and chronically ill. Juvenile rheumatoid arthritis has its onset prior to age of sixteen and sometimes goes through a complete remission over the period of several years. When it does not clear up, however, it continues to be a severe, chronic problem involving the entire body.

Hypertrophic arthritis gives an entirely different picture. This has been more commonly called osteoarthritis and is known also as degenerative arthritis, found more commonly in the older person. Yet, like many conditions afflicting the human frame, it can also be found in younger people. In this disease process there is generally no inflammation and no spreading or migratory type of joint involvement. Rather than a loss of calcium, there is a calcium buildup. An example of this is the so-called Heberden's nodes—a swelling and buildup of calcium about the base of the terminal bones of the fingers of both hands.

In osteoarthritis, there are calcific spurs and deformity of the joints, but never ankylosis (immobility and fixation of a joint), and rarely, if ever, the ulnar deviation of the fingers such as is found in atrophic arthritis.

There are, of course, other types of arthritis not quite so common. The arthritis associated with rheumatic fever, and those found with various inflammatory diseases, constitute the majority of this group. Gout might be listed in a separate classification. There is also a type of arthritis associated with trauma, which can be as difficult to correct as some of the others.

Concepts of Function

Physiological factors in the cause of rheumatoid arthritis are certainly different from those which bring about the condition we know as osteoarthritis. Thus it would not be surprising to find such a differentiation in the Cayce readings. The severity of atrophic arthritis, along with its poorer prognosis, leads one to suspect that the abnormal physiology is of a much deeper origin with much more profound ramifications.

There are certain basic causative factors, however, common to both conditions, as seen in the Cayce material. Poor eliminations and the associated condition, inadequate assimilations, seem to be part of the picture in nearly every condition of arthritis, no matter what type it may be. Apparently other abnormal functions within the body contribute to improper eliminations and direct the body down a course which brings either a mild or a serious condition which must be met.

In those cases which Cayce describes, treatment is seldom a simple procedure even when the person is not seriously ill. For instance, [4199] was told her problem originated from tautness of the muscles of the back and the nerves through the autonomic nervous system of the spine, which in turn produced lack of elimination through the skin or through the liver and kidneys. This then produced an autointoxication through substances which were picked up in the hepatic circulation. This condition of the blood supply created what is described as a "blood force" to the capillaries supplying the bursae and joint spaces of the lower extremities, thus causing a contraction in the lymphatic system of these sacs and hampering the action of the limbs themselves.

Cayce gave a reading for a man [1978] who was developing a tendency toward arthritis. There was a lack of liver activity as it is related to the function of the gall bladder, producing what Cayce called "solvents" for assisting in the assimilation of foods for the body. Perhaps his solvents are what we know as enzymes. This condition then apparently produced an inflammatory reaction which was carried through the blood, creating an inflammatory reaction in the extremities. Chemical imbalances in the body, lack of iodine in the bloodstream—these are mentioned as etiologic factors. One individual was told there was a crystallization of most of the foods that had certain elements or salts in them. His body was unable to deal with this and the crystallization then brought about the condition we call arthritis.

It should be noted, however, that Cayce did not limit his description of how a disease comes about by the ways in which the body's physiological functions are disturbed. In other cases, perhaps where the individual was able to deal with underlying causes more adequately, he explained that emotions which are chosen in interpersonal relationships have a major impact on how the body functions.

Rheumatoid arthritis, as mentioned earlier, is a different event in the human body. A fifty-seven-year-old man, [3363], was told he was experiencing rheumatoid arthritis as a "meeting of self." In the concept of karma, or "meeting oneself," the universal law states that what we are currently experiencing in our lives and in our bodies results from what we have done in times past, either during this incarnation or an earlier one in the earth. It's another way of saying what Paul said, "Whatsoever a man soweth, that shall he also reap." (Gal. 6:7)

This invariably involves one in his or her interpersonal relationships, for, as we pointed out earlier, it is not exactly what we have done as a life pursuit here as much as it is how we have performed in our relationships with others. Did we act in a kind, understanding, forgiving manner as a manifestation of the Love that God would have us live, or was it a self-serving attitude that said "This is what I want!"

Often rheumatoid arthritis is marked by the appearance of subcutaneous nodules. This man, [3363], was told the knots or cysts under the skin came about as a result of a "lack of proper distribution of energies that have been used in the body. Not wholly toxic conditions, but producing toxic conditions by their lack of proper elimination." This man, Cayce indicated, was suffering from lack of proper eliminations throughout his body, which brought about a crystallization of hormones in the circulation of the lymphatics. This created an incoordination between the lymph or superficial circulation and the deeper circulation. All the sympathetic nerves were under stress and strain so that in movements of the body, "these cry out for relief, as it were." There was a lack of proper assimilation as a part of the nerve disorder and disturbance.

In understanding the physiology in more everyday terms, we might see the development of some of these conditions described above as having their beginning in emotions that have been "stuffed" deep in the unconscious, but still acting through the autonomic nervous system to bring about derangement of the endocrine glands and their functions and an incoordination of the removal of the products of metabolism from the body, thus an intoxication or a "toxicity."

In a fifty-three-year-old woman, [5144], whose arthritis had progressed to the point of ankylosis, an unbalanced condition of the body as a whole weakened the resistance in the lymphatics and the emunctory (excretory) circulation through the extremities, especially in the bursae of the body. (Cayce described the bursae as those areas where lymph pockets are gathered in the regular functioning of the body.) *Dorland's Medical Dictionary* describes bursae as sacs filled with viscid fluid located in tissue where there would otherwise be friction. Thus Cayce's bursae would encompass the joint spaces, where most of the pathology in arthritis seems to be present.

Among persons with atrophic arthritis, assimilation was proposed as causing a glandular malfunction, as in [5150]. This brought about, in a secondary fashion, an infection, creating the arthritis. In another case, there was a lack of the glandular system's ability to reproduce itself. And in still another, the activity of the glands was given as the faulty mechanism and described as a karmic reaction. The glandular disturbance between the liver and the kidneys produced a suppression of elimination and an accumulation in the extremities, which is described as an arthritis tendency in still another case.

Memories of past lives are to be found in the endocrine glands of the body, somewhat expectedly, since our difficulties in life are nearly always emotional and traumatic. And the emotions have their origin and their dwelling place in these same glands. Cayce refers to the glands and the circulation, the eliminations, lymphatics and the nervous system as the areas where arthritis has its beginning.

The endocrine glands, you see, are closely related to the cardiovascular system through the hormones they supply to the bloodstream. Each of these glands, too, is a neurohormonal transducer, which means they are

deeply involved in both the hormones distributed to the
rest of the body and the nervous system as a whole. This
will be elaborated on later in another chapter, but it
helps to explain why the emotions, which live in the
glands, have deep relationships with the mind and the
body—each cell of the body

Hindered nerve reflexes, depression of the ganglia
coming about from poor assimilations and causing improper lymph function, and incoordination of the activity between the liver and the kidneys—all of these were
also pointed out as elements in the etiology of arthritis.

From the various functions which are seen to be abnormal, one begins to piece together part of the causative mechanisms seen in these psychic readings.
Disturbed elimination from any cause, certainly, seems
to be the primary abnormality of function. When there
are glandular disturbances, it seems more likely that a
rheumatoid condition should result, since glandular activity is so closely related to overall organ balance and
function, and in the Cayce readings the glands are seen
as the mediator of that balancing force which we know
as karma. Improper assimilation often comes about before or after the eliminations are disturbed, and the
nerve function from the ganglia of the autonomic nervous system is involved in the abnormal physiology.

The readings would likely imply that the development
of arthritis is an attempt on the part of the ligaments
and the joints themselves to meet the needs of the system poisoned by drosses present in the bloodstream.
The lymphatics, then, and the lymphocytes, with all
their resources, are unable—in conjunction with the
hormones—to bring about (what Cayce calls) a full co-
agulation or a building up of tissue from energy, a recon-
struction, in a sense, of the cells of the body.

Thus, the type of arthritis is determined to a great extent by the derangement of function prior to the onset of improper eliminations. It is probably more closely associated with the hormonal disturbance in rheumatoid arthritis, while in osteoarthritis the body is better balanced in most of its activities and not subject to such functional imbalances as comes about in the atrophic manifestation of the disease.

From Another Viewpoint

Arthritis is probably the most common ailment of the human body, aside from the common cold, but it is probably less understood than most. And its name is poorly chosen. The dictionary defines arthritis as inflammation of a joint. But medically, we know arthritis often starts with a tenosynovitis. What does this mean? An inflammation or abnormal state of the tendon and/or its synovial sheath. Generally speaking, arthritis can act as an umbrella for a variety of conditions called bursitis, myositis, tendonitis, etc. Thus the bursa of a joint can be involved with inflammation, or a muscle or a tendon—or, in reality, any part of the body closely associated with a joint in its action. Strange, isn't it?

Physiologically, the basic malfunction in any of these structural areas comes about through the introduction of an irritation we call inflammation. It would seem rational, would it not, if we could eliminate the inflammation at any stage of the process and subsequently introduce a regeneration activity, the tissues would be returned to normal?

Some years ago, I did a study of rheumatoid arthritis with a number of patients, using several of the concepts in the Cayce readings intended to bring about some of these changes I just mentioned. The study did not bring about any significant information or full resolution of the problem in these patients, although there were some improvements noted, but in my research of the literature I found a report indicating I was indeed on the right track.

In this report, a woman who had severe and painful arthritis of the lower extremities was operated on. The doctors (Kammerer and Hoen) performed a lumbar sympathectomy on her as part of a research study. This procedure destroys the sympathetic nerve supply to the hip joint. Four years later, she was readmitted to the hospital for a synovectomy (removal of a synovial cyst) of the right elbow. A repeat X-ray was done on her right hip, and they found a "startling improvement" in the radiographic appearance of the hip, consisting of remodeling of the joint, improvement in the texture of the bone and an increase in the joint space.

These structural changes can only be called regeneration of tissues. The woman no longer had any pain in the joint, and it can be concluded the inflammation present in the hip joint prior to the surgery was eradicated by the procedure which cut out the sympathetic nerve supply to that area. Thus, the imbalance between the sympathetic and the parasympathetic portions of the autonomic nerve supply was corrected in a way that allowed regeneration to take place. Interestingly, the parasympathetic system is the portion of the autonomic which rebuilds the body during sleep. The sympathetic input was markedly decreased in its action through the surgery, making the parasympathetic dominant in that area.

We don't know, of course, what sort of diet the woman followed. Nor do we know how much she believed the therapy would heal her body. And we won't know whether she was a woman dedicated to prayer and meditation, and whether or not she had others praying for her. These are factors Cayce talked about in the healing of any disturbance. What we do know, however, is that the surgery created a different environment within the woman's body: the inflammation stopped, and regeneration of the tissues took over and returned the ailing portion of the body back toward normal.

I knew, of course, that every person who was treated with a lumbar sympathectomy did not respond as this woman did. But in her case, why did the procedure work? The major factor was relief from the sympathetic input. So we need to explore the meaning of the sympathetic nervous system activity.

Answers might be found in many of the textbooks of neurology or neuroanatomy. The star performers in the sympathetic nervous system are the coeliac (solar) plexus and the adrenal glands. The adrenals are called the fight/flight glands and prepare the body for a threat of any kind, no matter what one understands to be a stress, an invasion or a danger. What the body sees as a risk, a peril, a menace, anything which puts the body as a whole into jeopardy activates the sympathetic nervous system immediately and creates a whole system of changes. One major alteration comes in the blood supply, which directs the major portion of the blood flow away from the organs of assimilation and elimination and orders the blood flow toward the muscles, tendons, and joints of locomotion or movement. Why this? To get the body either moving immediately away from the threat or preparing to fight.

When neither flight nor fight comes about after this correction of the blood flow, the joints and tendons and muscles are overloaded with blood and hormones (coming from the adrenals) which were not used. And the result is a relatively toxic condition. If the stress is sustained (as in a job situation, for instance) then destruction sooner or later comes into play, since the body cannot take the toxins away fast enough without physical action, and the elimination and the assimilation are both hampered. Trouble arises and one of the results is called arthritis.

There are, of course, more factors involved here than can be easily and comprehensively brought into focus. Some individuals handle stress as an adventure, which they like, and the result of the internal changes are not associated with fear, but rather worked through, and the individual balances the "forces" of the body so that health comes about, instead of disease or dis-ease. Most of us, however, are not able to deal with difficulties that constructively, and this may be why probably half of the population of the United States or more show some signs of this physiological series of events which end up with the tag "arthritis."

The Body Often Responds to Simple Measures

Because of my work with the Edgar Cayce concepts of healing, a woman named Lily wrote me a letter telling me about her experiences with simple healing procedures. Her brother-in-law had been scheduled for surgery on his arthritic right middle finger "to scrape off" the crystals formed there which were giving him much pain. Before the date of the surgery arrived, he followed his sister-in-law's advice and rubbed castor oil on his finger every day. Two weeks later, when he went to see his surgeon before being operated on, his arthritis and the pain were gone and no surgery was needed. Lily was happy about this incident, but had a more important story to tell me:

"I have a neighbor/friend who is in her eighties. She called me about the two middle fingers of her hand which were locked and unable to be moved—and had been that way for years. Her thumb at that time was twice its regular size and the little and index finger were giving her so much pain that she was unable to move them. And she was often crying with the pain. I didn't think it would be possible to unlock the fingers or correct the thumb because they were so bad, but I knew castor oil was very helpful.

"In order to get her hands active, we got her a container for a foot bath and used a pound of Epsom salts which we dissolved in hot water. Then we had her bathing her feet for a half hour each evening, all the time pressing, rubbing or massaging her feet. Then she was to wrap her hands in cloth saturated with castor oil, and apply a castor oil pack (with a heating pad on top) to her abdomen. She called a couple of days later saying the hands were no longer hurting her, and she was continuing the treatment. I wanted to document the progress, so went over to her place two weeks later with my camera.

"To my immense surprise, those two fingers were unlocked and she was making quilts. She said she used the foot bath with water as hot as she could stand it for the time I stressed, then put the castor oil pack on her stomach with a heating pad and wrapped her hands with cloths soaked in castor oil and put on rubber work gloves.

"Today the fingers are still unlocked and she is still making quilts. However, sometimes the fingers ache so she just gives them another treatment, and she is happy again."

Healing Comes in Strange Ways

Some years ago, a letter came across my desk reporting on a healing experience which seems to be one of a kind. This is Ralph's story:

"In 1957, I was found to have arthritis in both knees, which became very painful and was accompanied by much calcification in the joints. X-rays were taken, which confirmed the diagnosis. My doctor told me he could remove the calcium, but could not replace my kneecaps. I vetoed the surgical idea, but was told then that I would have to live with the pain, which I did until 1968.

"Later on that year, I experienced a time of what I can only call cosmic enlightenment in which I asked for and received the 'power to love' all of God's creatures. This also took away my desire to judge or condemn any fellow human being, regardless of behavior, creed, color, sex, or any other qualification.

"In February 1969, I discovered (quite by accident) that the grinding noise and pain in my knee joints had disappeared. My arthritis was gone and has never come back."

Ralph's experience reminded me of a comment that I heard attributed to Cayce: that there's as much of God in a teaspoonful of castor oil as there is in a prayer! We need to remember this. With each of us being body, mind, and spirit, we have the opportunity to understand better that meditation, prayer, change of consciousness toward the Christ and the Universal Forces can create healing as well as a medication, the knife, and something as simple as castor oil. We really are one at a deep unconscious level, and it is always well to recall to mind that we are indeed wonderful creations formed in the image of God. When God is at work through us in the healing process, anything good can happen.

The Touch of the Healing Hand

It was many years ago that Dolores Krieger, a Ph.D. in nursing, lectured on what she called "Therapeutic

Touch" at one of the Annual Medical Symposia spon-
sored by the A.R.E. medical clinic. She had been teaching the nurses at New York University School of Nursing
how to use their hands in a loving way to help bring healing to those for whom they were caring. Dr. Krieger's
workshop was so much in demand at the Safari Hotel
that we had to hold it outside on the spacious lawn near
the swimming pool.

Today it is difficult to find anyone who does not appreciate and understand the value of touch to the ailing
or to the healthy human being. Medical schools still have
a problem with the use of healing touch because of their
worship of what is called medical science. We have not
yet, you see, found out exactly how to do double-blind
studies of healing energy, which is extremely difficult to
measure. And medicine today still needs measurements
and proof to believe something good has happened to
the physiology of an individual human body. It should
be noted, however, that attitudes in medicine as a whole
have been changing for the better.

Wynne Christie spoke at the A.R.E. Congress in June
1994 on Therapeutic Touch. She lectured on the findings
and assumptions, the effects and the phases of treatment, correlating them with many Edgar Cayce readings
that explain how energies emanate from the hands and
how we can bring, in that manner, healing to the human
body.

Krieger postulated that the healing relationship is
based on a transfer of "life energy" present in all living
organisms. In health, this energy flows in, through, and
out of us in abundance, but in states of disease it is
blocked, disturbed, impaired, or depleted. Yet all individuals have an intrinsic ability to heal or to assist other
people to heal themselves.

Therapeutic Touch is now practiced by thousands of

professionals and lay people. There are also more than eighty colleges and universities in the United States teaching one form or another of this healing method in graduate and undergraduate nursing programs. What does it do, this energy? Those who are now professionals in the field have observed that it elicits a strong relaxation response: the breath slows, the blood pressure drops, muscle tension relaxes. As a result, anxiety level is reduced. With the decrease in anxiety, pain levels decrease. Changes occur in the patient's perception of pain, and one's natural healing ability is enhanced. Studies have shown that hemoglobin levels are raised; cell regeneration is speeded up; and the immune system is stimulated to perform more effectively.

Life Energies in the Cayce Readings

Edgar Cayce indicated we influence another person directly with this life energy when we sit or stand next to them. And he had much to say about touching. But his words always seemed to be directed internally; he saw what was going on with the life energy inside the body, and as it was directed outwardly. For instance:

Each atomic force of a physical body is made up of its units of positive and negative forces, that brings it into a *material* plane. These are of the ether, or atomic forces, being electrical in nature as they enter into a material basis, or become *matter* in its ability to take on or throw off. So, as a *group* may raise the atomic vibrations that make for those positive forces as bring divine forces in action into a material plane, those that are destructive are broken down by the raising of that vibration! ... So does the *entity become* the healer. 281-3

Cayce also noted that:

... this consciousness of [Christ's] presence must
be the basis of all healing ... 281-3

And also:

For all healing, mental or material, is attuning
each atom of the body, each reflex of the brain
forces, to the awareness of the Divine that lies
within each atom, each cell of the body. 3384-2

So it seems the energies coming from the hands of the
healer are without question the forces of the Divine flowing through those hands. And the energy then reacts
within the recipient in such a manner as to change the
vibrations—the attuning of the Divine within the living
tissues of a body to Creative Energies—and bring about
a divine experience within the cells and the atoms of the
body. Cayce speaks about these energies as available to
any who wish to be part of the healing process.

So, How Does the Average
Person Respond to This Power?

In my own experience, I have always—since discover-
ing the Cayce material—tried to touch the patient
while listening to his or her heart or chest, taking the
blood pressure, helping the patient to get up on the ex-
amining table or to sit down again in the chair. And I invariably give my patient a hug. That could be the medical
doctor's approach to use of the healing touch. The osteopath, the chiropractor, and the massage therapist all
have an advantage in this field, because they already are
using their hands to manipulate the muscles or joints or

adjust the infirmities of the body.

Every person on the planet can touch another and send with it those feelings of love and concern, and both will benefit from the touch. This particularly helps in the instance of arthritis, as hugs soothe the emotions of both individuals, the hugger and the huggee. And the soothing touch renders an acid condition of the body more toward an alkaline state, and better immune function.

Jesus was able to touch a person who was ill and instantaneously the patient was healed. He used His voice when He commanded Lazarus, who was dead, to arise. And he did. Jesus' robe had enough of His energy in it that the woman was healed of "an issue of blood" when she touched the robe. He used mud and spittle to bring sight back to the blind; and the power of faith He recognized in the centurion to heal his servant's son, who lay extremely ill at home.

In fact, all living human beings, the earth itself and those mineral, vegetable, and animal forms which it has brought forth are made up of atoms, nothing but energy brought into material manifestation. Eric Butterworth, a Unity minister, once said, "Materiality is consciousness outforming itself." We are using energy no matter what kind of healing we are considering or using, and consciousness is always the source.

Aching Joints and Muscles

Many of us have never been diagnosed with arthritis, but sprained ankles, dislocated shoulder joints, injuries to the knees or back or various muscular groups, whether brought about by sports activities or simple missteps in the daily living process are often related. How to ease them or give permanent relief becomes the challenge. Massages, manipulations, electrotherapy, or medicines are our most common remedies, but it is always helpful to recognize that Cayce frequently offers insights which give us a different perspective on what is transpiring when healing occurs. This reading reminds us:

Remember, mechanical (osteopathic) adjustments, like even properties as may be taken of the medicinal nature, are only correctives—and *nature* or the *divine* force, does the healing! 1467-9

Some time ago, an A.R.E. member told me about his bout with aching joints and muscles, brought about by strenuous work when he was not used to it.

"After three years of pushing nothing more demanding than a pencil, five continuous hours of swinging a hatchet and pushing a bow saw against a fallen tree left my right elbow strained and extremely sore. Rubs, heat, and the loving ministrations of friends for over a month didn't release the jaws that now clamped my arm painfully from wrist to shoulder. I could not stretch my arm to full extension at all, nor raise it over my head. The mere attempt left my hand shaking as if palsied, and my body in a fit of sweating."

B.J. listened to a friend who worked at a health spa as a masseuse and who introduced him to an oil that in her experience was very helpful. It was one of Cayce's formulations including coal oil, mineral oil, olive oil, witch hazel, tincture of benzoin, and sassafras oil. (See *An Edgar Cayce Home Medicine Guide,* A.R.E. Press, 1982, p. 85.)

He massaged his arm and shoulder with the oil several times that afternoon and evening. By nightfall, half of the pain was gone. The next morning he could extend his arm almost completely with only a minimum of trembling in his hand and almost no pain. He was able to raise his arm over his head for the first time in weeks. Continuing the applications of the oil, he gained complete freedom of movement for his arm with no shaking of his hand. His pain was gone.

More Understanding

There are many forms of arthritis. The early manifestations, however, may be simply stiffness of the joints of the body, slowness of walking, sometimes aching in the joints. It may be diagnosed as bursitis or tenosynovitis, a low back problem, difficulty in neck movement, or simply "My body is hurting." Many symptoms, certainly, act as a prelude to what may later develop into osteoarthritis if no preventive measures are brought into play, reversing the condition.

Cayce's view of the inner workings of the body frequently takes in the workings of the lymphatics, the blood supply, the essential organs of the body, the neurological systems, as well as the actual structural portions of the body. And it is different in each individual.

Improvement of the diet, exercise, and improved elimination can often prevent this kind of arthritis. But never discount the potentials of the human being when it comes to healing. Faith, enthusiasm, massage, local treatment, changes in consciousness or in the way one thinks—all of these can turn one from illness to health. And many have done just that.

A man who experienced this kind of benefit—in his own creative manner—was Lawrence Wolitz of Martinsville, Virginia. We corresponded about his problem and he gave me the following "informal update" because his condition had improved so dramatically.

"Background: My right shoulder became painful—could not raise my arm above my shoulder; many sleepless nights; could not reach my handkerchief in my back pocket. My physician's diagnosis: bursitis, for which only some painkiller pill or shots were offered. I did neither. I applied castor oil packs for three months to the point of seeming stability of the condition with pain and discomfort greatly reduced.

"Whereupon, I wrote to you, and you suggested peanut oil rubs and infra red heat. Imagine my total surprise when upon one treatment I was able to raise my arm overhead! I keep up the treatment about twice a week. My shoulder may not be totally cured, though I'm hardly aware of the pain.

"Now, please note this: within a week after beginning the oil rubs, I awakened one morning with what seemed to be a severe cramp at the back of my right knee. In the following days the pain and cramped condition caused me to limp heavily. I then realized that it was not your normal cramp. I began to apply peanut oil and heat to it and now it also is under control, and I can walk normally."

Injuries of one sort or another can often predispose to arthritis or those symptoms which are often associated with arthritis. Richard relates a history of back problems stemming from a football injury suffered in 1964:

"I had surgery in 1966 and again in 1980 to remove parts of a crushed disc. In November 1987 I hurt my back again, and went to a chiropractor for an adjustment. I was out of work for several days, showed improvement, and returned to work. I started suffering sciatic pain a few weeks later which radiated down my left leg. For the next month, I visited the chiropractor four more times, had bed rest, electrical stimulation, Motrin®, aspirin, Tylenol®, ice, heat, massage, etc. Nothing seemed to help. In fact, the pain got worse.

"I am a member of the A.R.E., and my wife and I both

enjoy reading the Edgar Cayce material. My wife was reading your book about the castor oil packs the same day I had given up and had gone to a regular doctor. The doctor set up an appointment for me with a neurosurgeon for the next day. The evening before I went to the surgeon, Ellen applied a castor oil pack for one hour to my lower back. I felt some relief, but was still in a lot of pain. At this point I was convinced that surgery was the only course left. The surgeon examined me, set up a myelogram, blood work, and X-rays. My wife continued applying castor oil packs and heat.

"After several days of castor oil packs and a few doses of olive oil by mouth, the pain was completely gone. I cancelled all appointments. After a two-day break, Ellen applied the castor oil packs for three more nights. I have not had any recurrence of back pain or sciatic pain.

"I am convinced that I have experienced a miracle and I am thankful to my higher powers, my wife's persistence and faith, and the information provided in your book at just the right time."

I'm sure the effect in Richard's case was physiological—we do not know enough about miracles to think of them as anything except universal laws bringing about changes whose mechanisms we do not yet understand. Although for Richard it was a miracle. On the other hand our limited research in the readings on the use of castor oil packs showed that relief of pain was described in eighteen cases; reduced inflammation in nine instances; increased relaxation in eight; and reduced swelling in four readings. All of these responses help in the basic relief of the underlying cause of arthritis.

4

How Can the Physical
Body Renew Itself?

ᘖ

In an earlier chapter, correction of your diet became the very first step in bringing about healing of your arthritis. If you have already taken some of those ideas to heart, your healing—your renewal—has already begun. But, as I mentioned earlier, there's lots more to come.

Arthritis does not come from external conditions. There has to be a problem inside the body or we do not gain the right to say, "I have arthritis!" Two people may eat exactly the same diet. One develops arthritis, the other flourishes in good health. The same two people may disagree about whether the air conditioning should be turned on. One may become chilled and develop creaky joints. The other may love the cold weather. In other words, the cause of arthritis is always found within the human body. Likewise, the correction for the same disorder must be found where the problem had its origin—within.

Most often, we take the cells of our bodies, our glands, organs, and even the systems of our body for granted. They are working okay, it appears, so we give them no further thought. However, when we develop aches and pains that seem to be inside, we become a bit apprehensive and wonder what is going on.

It's helpful to recognize these symptoms are, for the most part, only signals indicating the functions of these structures inside our beings have simply fallen a bit below the norm. And the norm is a state of good health. All we need to do, then, is reestablish a state of normalcy. If we do this early on in the game, while we are still in moderately good health, we may prevent arthritis and never even know what we prevented.

This, of course, is true for the common cold, cancer of the lung, for instance, and all the infirmities that might be found in between. A fundamental rule of balance lies at the core of this kind of reasoning. Each cell and each gland of the body have consciousness, as do the organs and systems. All have a consciousness of their own. Like people, they need to cooperate with each other in order to have peace. Then, when there is peace, all these structures coordinate with each other and bring about a state of balanced health.

We find, then, what is needed when one has arthritis is not a medication to take away the calcium buildup or to remove the pain. What is needed is therapy aimed at enhancing the functioning of the lungs, the liver, the kidneys, the heart and the circulation, as well as the entire nervous system. Not to *make* the functioning better, but to *awaken* and aid these structures to regain their normal activities.

The diet that has been suggested has several purposes. First, it aids the function of assimilation of foods. It makes for better and more coordinated use of the acids and enzymes in digestion, while allowing the stomach to produce the normal amount of mucus. The mucus protects the lining of the stomach while the acids and enzymes do their job of readying some of the foods for further processing.

The diet also aids in elimination of "used and refused forces," as Cayce describes the products of metabolism and the leftovers of the food products that are never used, nor needed. A large green salad at noon renders the body much more alkaline and most often prevents constipation. Eight glasses of water a day helps clean the urinary tract.

Such a diet stimulates the liver to work more normally in its detoxification of substances that need its efforts, and in its assignment to take part in elimination of metabolites. The diet also keeps the body tissues slightly on the alkaline side, which accentuates the ability of the immune system to rebuild the body—part of its function.

With all the wonderful happenings taking place inside the human body, we know our diet has more functions that are important than only those few I've mentioned.

What further steps do we need to take, then, in moving toward healing the body's arthritis? Especially now that we have established a good diet as the beginning point.

Next, let's help the skin eliminate by using Epsom salts baths. The skin, you know, is another of the organs of elimination.

Exercise! Don't stop too soon. Help the lungs as they not only aid the eliminations but also bring into the body substances necessary for life—oxygen, and other important, but hard to detect, properties the body needs.

Use castor oil packs on the abdomen. This helps the

immune system to function more normally.

Iodine: to help in gaining a better balance in and among the seven endocrine glands, which we call the seven spiritual centers. Cayce gave readings for the chemist who wanted to make a less toxic iodine preparation, which he called Atomidine.

Dreams: make a habit to recall, record, and study them for inner knowledge, and to discover important past-life experiences or tendencies. They also give us insight into possible karmic difficulties, waiting to be met creatively.

Visualization, biofeedback techniques: to aid the mind in taking an active part in the healing process.

Work with attitudes and emotions—group or individual, with emphasis on the insights to be gained, the negative aspects of the unconscious mind that need to be let go of, and the need to meet God within His holy temple, which is your own body.

Healing by touch: This involves treatments by the masseuse/masseur or the osteopath, the chiropractor, or simply the hug you may give or receive.

Prayer and meditation: to make for a closer attunement with the Divine, which leads one to develop a more health-producing lifestyle.

Consider joining a study group of some sort that will help each individual to apply concepts of soul growth and healing in daily life.

Each of the above ten steps (diet has already been addressed) obviously needs to be looked at in greater depth than we have shown above. Each has its place in helping the body to regain its normal status. Each is part of the whole picture. Thus some have already been explored to an extent.

It is always useful to see things from a different perspective. When we look at life from the standpoint of our being eternal beings, experiencing the earth each time for soul growth, we find it necessary to see each experience as an opportunity, an event we have, in a very real sense, designed ourselves so we can truly gain something eternal and beneficial out of the experience. This means we treat the whole of life as an adventure, a series of happenings that shapes our lives and makes each step of the journey a joyful consequence of our search. We might call it a joyful expectancy that must be kept on the part of every desire to be healed. A healing attitude is as necessary as any application we may make. Cayce talked about this quality in many ways, pointing out several times that all healing comes from the Divine within, and it becomes necessary to change one's attitude and let the life forces become constructive and not destructive if healing is to come about. The selection that follows is helpful in looking at our own feelings, our own attitudes:

As to the mental attitude: Be good for something. Not that we are questioning the purpose or the ideals of the body, but who healeth thy diseases, who forgiveth thy iniquities? These truths ye must trust in, actively; not merely passively but actively— holding no thought of grudge of any nature toward anyone. And you will find you will be a lot better. 3363-1

The remaining nine steps will be found here and there in the following chapters of this book, but will be easily recognized.

Regeneration—Renewing the Body

We pretty well understand that it is not the surgeon, but our body that really does all the healing after we undergo surgery or recover from an accident. Seldom, however, do we recognize the simple healing of a surgical wound is entirely different from the regeneration that happens when two segments of a fractured bone are splinted and healing starts. The body does its somewhat miraculous work in restoring the bone to its original condition, with no trace of a scar. Scarring is one thing, regeneration another.

In regeneration, the tissue is influenced by electrical impulses introduced by the body itself or from outside sources. The result can be, as in the salamander, the rebuilding of an extremity or a part of it, the rebuilding of the liver or, as mentioned above, the rebuilding of the bone. All tissues which are regenerated are restored back to the condition that existed prior to the injury or disease producing the loss. There are rules which must be followed in order to bring about the regeneration, but the end result is renewal or healing. This is what can happen in arthritis or almost any condition of the body lacking full health.

Much has been learned about regeneration in recent years, but it has been going on inside the body since the very beginning. If the human body is kept in balance internally, there is literally no age limit that it may not attain to. Information has been available for years that tells us all of the body tissues are replaced every seven years, atom by atom, some more quickly than others.

In arthritis, for instance, calcium deposits in joints can be removed—either instantly or over a period of time, depending on what happens inside the body with the energies involved. Loss of normal joint tissue in the hips of someone with rheumatoid arthritis can be rebuilt back to normal. The process, of course, is not simple and all parts of the human being are involved one way or another.

There is an energy pattern permeating the physical human body which the body and its cells follow in this process of rebuilding. The pattern is best known as the "soul body" for lack of a better term and is the eternal part of each of us.

In life as we know it in the earth, a single cell is born of the union of the sperm and the ovum in the mother's womb, developing into a structure during the amazing explosion of life that takes place in utero. Toward the end of pregnancy—or sometimes shortly after birth—the soul then enters the infant's body to become one with it during all the years the individual lives this incarnation. And the soul, with all of its memories and habits, weaknesses and strengths acquired in previous lifetimes, has a major role to play in building, shaping, and individualizing the body and the personality of the child and ultimately the adult.

A human being, then, is part spiritual and thus eternal; part physical and thus limited in nature. But we as souls are created in the image of the Divine and have within us the capability to regenerate any part of our body. Even when it seems death has come, the soul can come back and the individual (body, mind, and spirit) can continue to live.

The story of Lazarus (from the Bible) is different from what is called today a near-death experience (NDE) mainly in that Jesus, while He was here on the earth, called the soul back. He had the power to do so. In a near-death experience, as we currently know it, the soul of an individual who is apparently dead is given an opportunity while in the spiritual dimension to return back to what we call the land of the living. Sometimes he or she may not choose to return, but simply to be sent back by directing forces in the spiritual realm having the authority to do so. When the person returns, he or she often

remembers what happened on the other side.
Life may be understood to be vested in the soul body,
which leaves the physical body when one "dies," but always is the vehicle for remembering at an unconscious
level the experiences and happenings of past lives, as
well as events that happen to us in the present lifetime.
Through the life force in the soul body, healing or regeneration can come about in any part of a physical
body, restoring it to its original form. This is the story
Edgar Cayce presented to those who would listen many
years ago.

I've seen individuals, however, in our residential program who have been afflicted with severe illnesses who
did not respond to what seemed to be the appropriate
therapy suggested in the readings. I have asked myself
"Why?"

In the Cayce material there was a woman [1472] who
was being given her fourteenth reading. She was asking
why she was not being healed. Cayce's response was interesting for a number of reasons, complicated—but
worthwhile considering since it sheds light on the nature of healing, as well as providing the reason why it was
not occurring in this instance. The following material
from the reading, and my analysis of what was being
said, in my language, helped me to understand better
why it was that healing did not come. This lady asked to
be told "why I received no help." Cayce's answer:

Because they didn't do what was indicated to be
done! It was not always the fault of the body, [1472].
Mostly it was because of the manner in which administrations were made by others. These as we
find are the faults, if faults they be. 1472-14

In this first paragraph, Cayce pointed out that most

likely there were no real faults to be found here. In his readings, he often said, "magnify the virtues, minimize the faults." But the problem was in the manner others about the patient were applying the therapies. This means, I am sure, their attitudes and their feelings were involved as well as their interpretations as to how the therapies should be done.

It is not meant that information given through this channel should be interpreted as being infallible, but these are the conditions existent as viewed from the condition of the individual entity. 1472-14

In the second paragraph, he was merely reminding them that the information he was reporting was the inner conditions present in the individual for whom he was reading, and probably—as was indicated later on, had to do with the spiritual forces—the God-force within and the balance within her as far as the spiritual-mental-physical relationship was concerned.

The interpreting of the information in the minds of others, as well as the manner in which the individual entity is influenced by others—by their material or physical knowledge, does not imply that the information given is incorrect. But it does imply that if these are met under certain other administrations, and done in the same manner and attitude that the information may be given, there may be produced a oneness—and [a] response in its own kind. 1472-14

The first sentence in the third paragraph needs to be read directly; it tells us the woman is influenced heavily by those around her and they are probably not interpreting clearly the readings given in the past intended to be helpful, and leads the reader to understand the information given is correct. But, interestingly, if her care under other kinds of treatments is to be done in the same attitude of helpfulness and loving care as is present in the reading, there may be produced a oneness and a healing result. The attitude is more helpful than the method—this seems to be the lesson from this part of the reading.

Here, for this body, as we find—and as we have indicated—there are disturbances in the lymph circulation, especially in the soft tissue of face and head. The antrum, the frontal and the inner area has shown infection, from the congestion and a general catarrhal condition. These arise from many sources, but from long-standing have begun to be of a constitutional nature. 1472-14

The fourth paragraph of the reading simply indicates what Cayce saw to be present in the face and head. The causes are multifaceted, apparently, and Cayce did not elaborate on what they were.

This does not imply, then, that these are incurable; but, as is the influence in *all* healing, whether the administration be purely suggestive, of a vibratory nature, from the laying on of hands, or by the spoken word, the administration of medicinal properties or even the use of means to remove diseased tissue, we find that the same source of individuality in the cause must be attained. That is, that which has been dissenting in its nature through the physical forces of the body must be so attuned to spiritual forces in itself as to become revitalized. 1472-14

This paragraph, perhaps, is most helpful in pointing out how the Cayce readings take the position that it is the elimination of warring or rebelling, "dissenting" forces within the individual that needs to be set aside in obtaining a healing. The method of working with the patient, however, may be any one of a number of procedures: suggestion, vibratory measures, laying on of hands, the spoken word, medicines, or surgery. The patient in this case—in order to be revitalized—must take that rebellious nature and attune those energies to her spiritual source, or those "spiritual forces" in herself.

As to what is that necessary influence to bring about curative or healing or life-giving forces for that individuality and personality of the individual with same, as related to the spiritual forces, may be answered only within the individual itself. For, no source passes judgment. For, the spirituality, the individuality of the God-force in each entity's combined forces, must be its judge. 1472-14

Cayce pursues the subject in this last paragraph and indicates the woman knows what has been blocking her progress. She knows within herself what influence is necessary to bring about curative or healing or life-giving forces. And this, undoubtedly, is the change needed in the previously mentioned "dissenting" attitudes that might then bring the body to an attunement with the Divine.

Reviewing the above material, in retrospect, my comments may be as difficult to understand as the advice Cayce gave this woman to consider in her reading. Yet, it seems clear that emotions are a part of the healing process, part of the regeneration that must come about. The emotions, of course, have their home in the endocrine glands, and we can deal more extensively with this subject later on in the book.

One thing seems clear, however: Our interpersonal relationships play a heavy role in how we fulfill our destiny or our purpose this lifetime. These relationships always bring about an interaction between our soul nature and the way we live. We want to be loving in the way God seems to direct us to be, based on how we understand the meaning of "God is love." Then, the endocrine glands take that desire and infuse our interpretation of what love might be into the bloodstream and the nervous system in the form of hormones and neurological impulses. Our material desires and leanings, however, play the part of the adversary and our higher sights are then, to an extent, clouded, resulting in turmoil or disturbance or out-and-out war instead of what we would deeply want to happen.

Thus, whether we have arthritis or a sore throat, the healing of the body is associated with the feelings we harbor and the manner in which we treat our fellow human beings. We cannot get away from the basic reason why we are here in the earth today.

Eliminations—Letting Go

The lymphatics are not usually perceived as eliminatory vessels, but, in actuality, they are exactly that. They provide the very first step in accepting the waste products from the cells of the body, along with the other products the cells create, and carry them to the thoracic duct, and from there to the venous system to travel through the lungs and the heart and then to be eliminated through the liver and the intestines, the kidneys, the lungs, or the skin. This is the body's way of getting rid of substances which are no longer needed in the human system. We need to let go of them. When we don't, constipation is the result. We can deal later with constipation as it relates to emotions and the mind. We must not forget that the common denominator of causes of arthritis is lack of proper eliminations.

In anatomy texts, the lymph system has been found to exist in all tissues of the body where there is any kind of a blood supply. We understand that where blood brings life to the cells, lymph exists to remove waste products from the cells.

The thoracic duct is an interesting structure, described in *Gray's Anatomy* as varying in length in the adult from thirty-eight to forty-five centimeters, extending from the second lumbar vertebra to the root of the neck, and having a number of valves, the last of which prevents venous blood from entering the duct as it empties into the angle of the junction of the left subclavian vein with the left internal jugular vein. The text further explains:

"The thoracic duct has a more complex structure than the other lymphatic vessels; it presents a distinct subendotheliel layer of branched corpuscles, similar to that found in the arteries; in the middle coat there is, in addition to the muscular and elastic fibers, a layer of connective tissue with its fibers arranged longitudinally. The lymphatic vessels are supplied by nutrient vessels, which are distributed to their outer and middle coats; and here also have been traced many non-medullated nerves in the form of a fine plexus of fibrils.

"The lymph is propelled by contractions of the vessel walls. The valves prevent the backward flow. The segments between the valves contract twelve to eighteen times per minute in the mesenteric lymphatic vessels of the rat."

The entire lymphatic system is part of the immune

system, supervised and directed by the thymus gland, and includes lymphatic structures such as the tonsils and adenoids, the Peyer's patches, the appendix, the lymph nodes throughout the intestinal system, the neck, axillae, groin, and other locations throughout the entire body. The liver and the spleen must also be included in this system, which is involved always with the balance between the acid and alkaline properties in the body.

Alkalinity in the System

An alkaline reaction within the body has been one of the best means mentioned in the Edgar Cayce readings to prevent colds, flu, and respiratory conditions of any kind. When your body is slightly alkaline in nature, you will have little likelihood of "catching" a cold. At the Clinic we have found this to be almost a standard for adequate protection

But why is this so? Perhaps the best answer is that the immune system works more efficiently in a slightly alkaline medium. The slightly elevated pH (hydrogen ion concentration) provides the normal environment for a healthy immune system. If the lymphatic stream becomes overacid for any reason, the immune system is not up to par; the body is then deficient in its defense overall and subject to invasion by viruses or bacteria already present in the body. The white blood cells and the immune system as a whole can no longer control them. And in arthritis, the buildup of substances normally excreted is increased, and the breakdown of the abilities of the immune system to restore normalcy causes other difficulties. So it is best to keep the pH of the tissues and the lymphatic stream slightly on the alkaline side.

How is this to be accomplished? First, eat those foods that are alkaline reacting in their nature—fresh fruits, fresh vegetables—and avoid too much meat, fat, fried food, starches, and sweets. All these are acid-reacting. Much of this is dealt with in chapter 2. Other causes can be found in our lifestyles. When we work in a sedentary occupation, our bodies tend to become overacid. We do not need heavy foods to sustain body activities requiring little physical effort. If we obtain too little sleep at night, there is not enough rebuilding and body tissues tend to become overacid, in a sense. When we are chronically involved in stress from home situations or work that is made stressful by supervisors or expectations to meet unreal deadlines—this is interpreted by the body and its endocrine system and emotions to be acid-reacting. Inability to adapt peacefully to life situations also brings about a similar imbalance between the acid and alkaline forces in the body.

Corrections for these disturbances can frequently come about from what some call attitudinal adjustments. Counseling, conscious choosing of a different approach to life, meditation. These are ways to help bring about a better acid-alkaline balance.

Lettuce as a Healer

From one of my correspondents comes a story about lettuce, and it has nothing to do with salads. Dorothy wrote that she has a new respect for this highly alkalinizing part of nature's bounty: "Every now and then I seem to develop an infection in my left arm. I know the arm is under stress, and swells a bit, ever since my mastectomy and removal of glands in my armpit. The infection seems to develop after I have a hangnail in my finger or an insect bite on the left arm. Usually I have had to seek out my doctor and get an antibiotic quickly, or I am in trouble.

"On one occasion my temperature had risen to over 103 degrees, and I was suffering. I had read in the Cayce material about lettuce being a blood purifier, and decided to try that as a remedy instead of some of the antibiotics which I still had left from my most recent trip to the doctors. I began with a small wedge of lettuce, chewed it up well before swallowing it, and then continued taking another small wedge every two or three hours. My temperature rose slightly. By evening, however, the infection had disappeared, the redness had gone, and my temperature was normal! I was convinced."

Was the blood purified? In the diet section of this book, lettuce is like the other greens in that it is an alkalizing portion of the diet. What happens in this instance inside the body physiology is another story. But whatever the final answer may be, whether purifier or alkalizer of the immune system, this lady's body was able to overcome the infection and for her the lettuce was better than her antibiotic.

Epsom Salts Baths

Edgar Cayce recommended Epsom salts baths frequently, especially to those who came to him seeking help for their arthritis. The benefit apparently comes from the effect of the salts on the surface of the body, plus the heating of the tissues of the body, increasing the circulation internally as well as externally. The internal effect, of course, would be the acceleration of the oxygen brought to the tissues of the body, but also the increased activity of the lymph drainage from the areas affected by the arthritis. The body temperature increases, as does the pulse. The result is a cleansing of the tissues troubling the body, and a gradual removal of the excess calcium buildup. In the case of rheumatoid arthritis, the effect of the increased circulation apparently—in the readings—increases the ability of the damaged areas to regain their normal status.

Most individuals will perspire rather profusely. Some will want to get out of the tub sooner than planned because they feel a bit uncomfortable. One of my patients, however, didn't understand my instructions to lie with his body immersed in the water as much as possible for fourteen or fifteen minutes and then, if he felt lightheaded, to sort of roll out of the tub onto the floor and rub himself dry with a bath towel. When he returned the next time, he told me he really felt good from taking the bath, although he thought forty-five minutes was a long time. He didn't need to roll out of the tub.

We usually tell patients to keep an ice bag handy to put on their heads if they have to sit up in the tub and feel light-headed. At times this will happen from the upright position draining some of the blood away from the brain. The ice bag helps.

Instructions for an Epsom salts bath:

Place two to four pounds of the salts in the bathtub. Start the hot water running in the tub and then climb in, immersing yourself as much as possible the whole time, stirring the water to dissolve the salts. Keep the water running hot until the tub is filled and your body is covered as much as the size of the tub will allow. Keep the water as hot as you can stand it.

Let the hot water continue to run as you stay in the tub for ten to fifteen minutes (or longer if your doctor advises). When you are ready to get out, shower first and then wrap yourself in a bath towel and lie down for one-half hour to let your body cool off.

How frequently should one best take such a bath? It
varies with different people. For some, twice a week is
best. For others perhaps once a week, or in rare instances
three or four times a week. It is always best to be consistent with a program you set out for yourself. Be patient
with yourself and, above all, persist in your attempts.

Exercise as an Aid

It is always helpful when taking a journey to reevalu-
ate what we are really doing. How does physical exercise
fit in with a spiritual journey? We have to remind ourselves we really are souls—spiritual beings—abiding for
the present time in a physical body. This is the perspective we need to claim as our own—a point of view that
needs to be revisited every now and then, so that our relationship with the body and the power of the mind are
recognized and applied as a reality now and involves—
at this time—the manner in which we exercise.

If we are truly one—body, mind, and soul (or spirit)—
then we need to treat each of these portions of our being
at their own level. That is, to exercise the physical body
in specific ways, not just to think about it or assume because we are spiritual beings that exercise is below our
spiritual level and thus not necessary. We need to take
into action our thoughts and beliefs about exercise. And
this, of course, is true about all the steps we might take
in the physical body about the healing of arthritis.

Edgar Cayce said frequently the best exercise is walking. All parts of our body associated with movement—
bones, joints, muscles, and tendons—need to be used
constructively. They need to be exercised. If we keep in
attunement with the God-Force vibrations, then the
problem is simplified. We are told that we are here to *do*
things, to be of service, to be helpful to others. As we

move in time and space to accomplish those tasks, our bodies move.

Our activity on Earth is expressed through our conscious muscular movements, whether they direct our voice, our hands or feet, or whatever. Indeed, if we had no ability to control these muscles, called striated muscles, we could not easily influence the world around us. Perhaps we could use our minds as tools and send out thought waves, but that is not using the physical body. The body-in-action is an overt manifestation of the individual life in this world and in this dimension, whether we are serving food in a restaurant or using a computer to help put another satellite into outer space. The conscious mind does these things in directing us to move in a specific manner.

It is the autonomic nervous system, however, that rules the internal organs of our bodies, directed for the most part by our unconscious mind. The condition of our organs and systems spells health or disease for the whole body, so it becomes important that the autonomic and the inner activity of the body be treated with thoughtful and constructive care. Exercise (along with the allied activities of manipulation and massage) has the responsibility of taking on this assignment.

Walking is the best exercise one might choose. Swimming and biking, as well as planned exercise routines, come close to being satisfactory alternatives to walking. Each of these, as well as massage and manipulation, works the structural parts of the body in its own specific way. The balancing effect brought about brings into the autonomic nervous system and the physiology of the functional body a better state of health. This, in turn, has its beneficial effect on the nervous system and the senses.

Exercise the body reasonably. Don't exercise so as to

cause stress or irritation to the body. Care gently for the
body is the best advice—don't overtax it.

About exercise, Cayce has this to say to one man, who
apparently was not following suggestions very well.
"Whether it's a mile or a step, do that which makes for a
better 'feel' for the body; getting into the open!" (257-
204) And the walking was often advised in the readings
to be done vigorously enough and long enough to bring
about a sweat on the body.

When the body is hampered by arthritic changes,
massage and/or gentle manipulation might be a better
choice than walking. Every choice is dependent, always,
on the individual and the person's needs.

A head-and-neck exercise can be used to bring about
greater flexibility in the cervical spine. If used regularly
over a long period of time, it will correct the rigidity
which sometimes comes about in certain types of arthritis (see Appendix). The hearing and visual acuity of the
eyes are both sharpened by using this exercise. In preparing oneself for meditation, the head-and-neck exercise has become widely used by A.R.E. members and
study group members throughout the world.

Any exercise which brings about more flexibility in the
spine will help the nervous system and the body as a
whole to maintain a better state of health. This is especially true of anyone who has arthritis.

Exercise Injuries

Exercise in one's own health maintenance plan—or
during participation in games—aids the body, but does
cause problems when injuries arise in the course of that
kind of activity. In a letter to me, Larry Miner contrib-
uted the following story of injury and, later on, the cure:

"I dislocated the end joint of my thumb playing handball, but it went back in quite easily after pulling it out a bit. The pain was not great while healing but prolonged—months, even—gradually becoming less and less tender.

"One day while skiing (below zero outside), I fell, but I don't know whether I hurt it then. I suspect it was the intense cold that started up the aching of the joint worse than at the time of the original injury. This time, however, after a few days, I tried a castor oil pack overnight for two or three nights. All discomfort and tenderness disappeared within those few days and has never returned."

Another one of my correspondents, Gregory Toothman, injured the medial meniscus of his right knee. He was unable to walk without crutches. His therapy program?

1. Castor oil packs every night on the knee for three months, all night long.

2. Twice daily massage of the affected knee under an infrared lamp using peanut oil as the oil of choice most of the time.

3. Bathe occasionally in a strong solution of Epsom salts (two pounds of the salts to a tub of water).

4. Occasional salt and vinegar packs to the knee.

He reported a gradual improvement, first leaving off the crutches, then increasing his activity and finally being able to run within the three-month period. No residual problems.

One wonders whether the knee would have healed that rapidly without such a regimen of therapy. However, most similar problems today would be corrected by surgery, or result in a problem knee when healing does finally come about. Greg's persistence, patience, and consistency paid dividends.

Jesse Gorman told me his story about his shoulders:

"In 1974, before I became acquainted with the Cayce concepts of healing, I suffered an accident. I developed a severe case of traumatic arthritis in both shoulders as a result of the accident, and a cervical spondylitis in the second and third vertebrae.

"I had surgery on one shoulder, and the orthopedic surgeon, the neurosurgeon, the orthopedic-neurosurgeon, and my Dr. Jones, who worked with the orthopedic surgeon, all agreed that I would never be able to use my arms to amount to anything, ever again. They were right—for seven years.

"After I began reading about the Cayce treatments, I began using peanut oil and an infrared lamp. In about four months, I noticed I had a little more range of movement in my arms and a little less pain.

"From then on, I slowly but steadily improved. Today my shoulders are almost healed and my neck is considerably better."

A sprained ankle is, in a very real sense, a kind of arthritis, traumatic in origin, but involving the welfare of joints. Gae Haefer wrote me about how she took care of her sprained ankle. She took her castor oil pack and placed it in her microwave oven for only thirty to forty-five seconds, because the pack gets hot quite fast. Then, placing it on her ankle and keeping it warm with a heating pad brought much relief to the injured part. She didn't tell me how long it was from the time of injury to the application of the pack, but everyone should know that immediate application of an ice pack to a sprained joint will do more to stop the bleeding than any other treatments. After half an hour or more, a heated castor oil pack has done wonders for alleviation of pain and swelling in simple sprains.

Massage, Manipulation, Body Work

The Cayce readings emphasize time and time again that full-body massage aids the functioning of the human body. Function is primarily based on the degree of electrical or nervous system coordination, not on the chemical changes within the body.

A paper published in the *International Journal of Sports Medicine* (1983) discussed the blood-chemistry changes in healthy males resulting from a massage given by a trained masseur. Although it does not touch on the neuroelectric effects, the article states that massage is recognized as having its most important effect through its sedative action, its reaction through certain reflexes, and its pumping action on veins and the lymphatics.

There are changes in certain enzymes, comparable to the effect on the body of heavy muscular work. This means liberation of these enzymes from muscular tissue. The hemoglobin is very slightly decreased, but basically no other changes were observed.

Neurologically, it is recognized that massage showers the entire nervous system with nerve impulses arising in the skin as it is stroked or massaged. It is also recognized that nerve impulses either allow the body to function normally or they create confusion.

A comprehensive discussion of massage was published in *The A.R.E. Journal,* Vol. V (Jan. 1970) by Mary Alice Duncan, R.P.T., who had studied the Cayce readings to see how they align with physical therapy. She pointed out how Cayce could "see" inside the individual cell, but, even better than that, "He could see the function of the cell in relation to the function of all other parts of the entity—physical, mental, and spiritual."

She pointed out how problems of the nervous system may be aided through the influence of massage to portions of the body where the problem may exist. And how important it is to have massages done by those who are wanting to be of service in this way. In the following reading, a long-term massage program was advised for a karmic problem for the mother and father as well as the child. The following advice was given:

> The massage may be done by anyone who is patient and persistent, but as indicated, do not attempt to delegate to someone else that which should be the privilege and the opportunity of the parents. Others may do it, even a little bit better, yet in mind, in body, in spirit, those who are to heal themselves in healing this body must do the applying. 3117-2

Cayce was always looking at the body as a whole, with all parts interconnected. We should remember that the nervous system—which is constantly worked on through the touch of the therapist on the skin of the patient—is involved in every action, every thought, and every emotion throughout the body. We are, indeed, a soul working through the physical body that takes us through this incarnation.

To gain a better understanding of how the functions of the body are always interrelated, another of the Cayce readings might be studied. It was given for a child who had an unidentified abnormality. After suggesting massage should be performed in the lumbar and sacral areas of the body, Cayce advised massaging also the feet and the soles of the feet. This, he said in reading 395-2, "will enable the body to soon gain that strength and an equilibrium sufficient to make for more activities in a different or better *position* for the body and the body-organs."

The massage, in this instance, was to feed impulses back to the spinal cord and the sacral parasympathetic plexus to build into the body a better ability to achieve balance, a greater strength in the muscles, and probably an improved functioning of the internal organs as a result of the change in body position to be acquired.

We cannot avoid the importance of massage to the body, perhaps as much through a healing touch as through the actual physiological-neurological changes elicited. Another bit of Cayce information may explain it better:

The "why" of massage should be considered: Inactivity causes many of those portions along the spine from which impulses are received to the various organs to be lax or taut, or allow some to receive greater impulse than others. The massage aids the ganglia to receive impulse from nerve forces as it aids circulation through the various portions of the organism. 2456-4

Cayce's position on manipulation—whether used by the osteopath or the chiropractor in those days—was always a positive one for the benefit of the body. In a very real sense, manipulation, massage, and exercise all bring activity to the living physical body and are necessary for the body's normal function. Today, both osteopathy and chiropractic are better known for their proven values than massage or simple exercise, although millions of Americans today avail themselves of this boon to their physical body. And the blessings to health and longevity cannot be overestimated

When one suffers from arthritis, however, there is need to choose between the kinds of help that would be most effective and most reasonable.

More on Castor Oil Packs

Roberta Williams, a massage therapist, is fascinated with castor oil and its value to the human body. I got this letter from her some time ago:

"I have been using castor oil on my clients now who have tight, knotted muscles in the back from stress. I apply a generous coat of the oil on the affected area, cover it with a sheet of Saran wrap and a towel, and cover the area with a warmed-up 'bean bag.' I make this by sewing a small terry-cloth towel into a bag containing about four cups of white rice (uncooked, of course). Before applying the rice pack, I heat it in the microwave for five or six minutes. It retains its warmth for almost an hour.

"I leave the pack on while I massage the legs, and by the time I get to the back or shoulder areas, the muscles are warm and soft, responding to the massage much better. The castor oil has been absorbed, so I use my regular oil and finish the massage as usual. This moist heat treatment feels wonderful and seems to give the desired relief—at any rate, everyone on whom I have used these packs insists on having one of their own, so I tell them how to make it."

When planning activities to bring healing to the body, you should follow your common sense. We know, for instance, the immune system is vital to the rebuilding of the body as well as protecting all parts of the body from the world around us. So, let's do everything we can to strengthen the capacity of the immune system to do its assigned job.

Our research in the use of castor oil packs as reported in chapter 1 indicated for us that the application of castor oil as a pack over the liver and upper abdomen does indeed aid the immune system. So, let's use castor oil packs (see Appendix).

Some time ago, Lucille wrote me wanting to share some of her experiences with castor oil. This is her story: "When I was pregnant, I had to take vitamins. The iron made me badly constipated. I discovered if I rubbed castor oil all over the abdominal area before I went to bed, I'd have a normal bowel movement in the morning."

She now applies the remedy whenever she has diarrhea, constipation, or a simple belly ache. It doesn't seem to matter what's wrong, "the castor oil fixes it by morning. I sometimes use heat, but not usually."

Last year, Lucille's mother visited her, bringing with her a severe case of constipation. A self-prescribed enema only brought on the runs. Lucille said, "I finally convinced her to rub the castor oil on her abdomen. She refused to use heat. The next morning I would have sworn she had a personality transplant. The desired results were achieved! Also, for as long as I can remember, she's had extreme flatulence. But now she rubs the castor oil on every day and doesn't have that problem anymore. It's made such a difference in her attitude. She's so much more positive now."

Lucille's mother didn't even use a pack, but her attitude took a great turn for the better, and her intestinal tract appears to be more normal and balanced in its autonomic functions.

Castor oil packs are simple, yet effective means of helping the inner parts of the body to function more normally.

5

What Role Does the Mind
Play in This Journey?

〜

Let's look at one of our original concepts again. Our true beings, our souls, were created in God's image, and, as we understand it, were made up of spirit, mind, and will (or choice). We each were given life, manifesting as spirit in the soul body; we were fashioned with the gift of choice, so we could even deny we were actually created in the image of God. Or we could use the gift of choice to agree, and thus use our power of choice to direct our ways through our earth experience.

Too, we were made in the likeness of God in that we have a mind, which is a power, a strength, a means of doing whatever we have chosen to do. Our minds are creative, allowing us, whenever we find ourselves in relationships with others, to build toward harmony in our lives or to make turmoil and pain and havoc. We must remember, we can choose to build mansions, ships, bridges, computers, as well as tending to our primary mission: learning how to love God and our fellow human beings, wherever they may be throughout the earth.

One of the Cayce readings spoke to the purpose for which we were born:

> That God hath so willed that man should be free to choose should indicate for each individual his relationship to God, that may only be manifested in the manner the individual treats his fellow man. 281-60

While writing this particular portion of this book on Easter weekend, I did some research on the events of this season as described in the Cayce material in order to see how arthritis could be associated with what happened two thousand years ago.

Healing of the body, whether it be arthritis or heart disease, or whatever, is often a major episode in the life of that body. There is always a reason for it becoming part of our life. The primary reason we are faced with such a problem may be that we need to make changes in our direction so our actions will become more and more in harmony with God's will. Cayce talked about that, too:

> And *again* ye have seen, when to man's estate alone upon the cross, yea into the grave, all hope seemed abandoned, yet even as the inn could not contain His birth, neither could the grave contain His body; because of it *being purified,* in love, in service, in harmony to God's will. For, "Not of myself," saith He, "but the Father that worketh in and through

me do I bring thee health, do I bring thee hope, do I
bring thee the living waters." 1152-4

When we talk about changing our direction so that our
actions will become more and more in harmony with
God's will, we probably don't fully realize what this
means, since the answer lies in the mystic realm of the
unconscious mind, deposited there during events that
took place in a past life or a series of lifetimes. The above
reading, however, indicates that increased harmony au-
tomatically brings about healing of the body, the "health
... hope ... the living waters."

We create, always, whether it is in a loving manner
with a spouse or the hate engendered by deep disagreements that lead to anger. In these disagreements, we
might say, "I want my own way! I do not want to understand or forgive, I simply want to do things that are right,
according to what I see is the truth."

There is a slight problem here because the other person involved may be thinking the same thing and with a
full right to do so. In past lives, each has a different set of
experiences, and these become learned reactions from
the unconscious mind moving through us and telling the
world, "This is what I am and this is the truth."

So two individuals who are both living their truths
have disagreements because the truths are in conflict. A
few words from the sleeping Cayce helps us understand
this conflict: "For what is truth today may be tomorrow
only partially so, to a developing soul!" (1297-1)

In another instance, Cayce answered a question for a
young man about what different spiritual organizations
he should study. Cayce's answer adequately speaks to the
two truths that were in conflict in the story above:

These had best be studied in the light of that

which is desired to be attained by the body. For each, to be sure, in their sphere of activity, have some truth; but no finite mind has *all* the truth! For *truth* is a *growing* thing! 282-4

The two individuals living their truths could begin to deal with these clashes by choosing to adopt and nourish a position of listening to one another, and then talking about the differences to gain an understanding of the other's point of view. This produces amazing results at times and it boils down to a change of direction in our lives. Our actions then will become more and more in harmony with God's will. A choice! Part, at least, of the process of bringing healing to the body.

Some time ago, a woman in her thirties developed a headache that would not go away. She finally saw her doctor; she was given multiple medications that did not work, and she was referred to a neurologist. All of this with no significant help for her headache. She was finally sent to a neurosurgeon who did brain surgery on her because of certain findings that were interpreted to be a tumor of the pituitary.

Brain surgery was performed again with no diagnosis. Biopsies did not reveal any malignancy. Her headache persisted and it was always severe and unrelenting. A friend urged her to come to our Clinic because of the way we work with the Cayce concepts of healing. She started looking within and began to understand the kind of choices she had been making in her life. She then decided to come through one of our residential programs. Her marriage was rocky, her anger was easily set off, and her life was deteriorating. For years she had sought a deeper understanding of her spiritual life and now she was determined to get well.

She arrived in Phoenix, started the Temple Beautiful

residential program, and made the conscious choice to be open to everything that was going to happen. Her body was treated, of course, but it was her mind that manufactured dreams, and her dreams were, for her, truly amazing. She gained glimpses of some past-life experiences and insights into what was happening in her present life.

She was taught how to use biofeedback techniques to access her involuntary forces with her voluntary mind—that is, suggest to her body deep inside that it function in a more constructive manner. On the second night of her stay in the program, she decided to wake up the next morning free of the headache. Powerful use of the mind, associated with the ability to choose what she wanted to happen. She did, of course, wake up the next morning free of any sign of a headache. And the relief not only persisted, it entirely changed her life for the better. Her husband called to tell us that a new, loving woman stepped off the plane to enter into his life, and he was grateful.

I'm sure this young lady used her mind to make choices in some respect similar to another woman who was advised through one of Cayce's readings. She was confronted with difficult situations, and she wanted to know how she could be sure the decision she reached was from the Light and not from her own thinking. This is Cayce's advice—but whether she took it or not is not known:

As the body recognizes, there is the body-mind, the body-consciousness, there is also the inner consciousness or the soul-mind. Ask the question in self in the physical mind so it may be answered yes or no, and in meditation get the answer. Then closing self to physical consciousness, through the meditation, ask the same question. If these agree, go ahead. If these disagree, analyze the own self and see the problem that lies in the way. 5019-2

The Mind and Its Choices

A number of years ago, the idea of my considering any disease to be an adventure in consciousness or a spiritual journey had its inception. Several simple ideas caught my attention. One (and not necessarily the first) was found in Galatians 6:7: "Make no mistake about this: God is not to be fooled; a man reaps what he sows." Cayce said it this way: "What is meted must be met." We don't do anything in this world that impacts other people or the world around us without gaining the results, whether our actions create glory and happiness or simply reap the wild wind.

In thinking about my adventure in consciousness, I believe the Bible and Cayce were saying to me that I always (at the present time) experience what I have created, or sowed, somewhere in the past either in this lifetime or in an earlier one. If it is an illness, then there is a cause relating the illness, through the body physiology and emotions, to the Cayce concept that all illness is sin lying at my doorstep.

In some manner all the accidents, all the illnesses, all the difficulties we experience have their origin within our own beings, our own actions, whether in this life or another. In some cosmic manner, this is reality, whether we like it or not. Karma is the name given to these ideas—if you throw a ball against a wall, it will come back to you. An ancient idea, true, but always there.

Another bit of the jigsaw puzzle was the simple statement in Genesis 1:27: "So God created man in his own image." Putting logic into biblical material, we know God is a spirit (and eternal), so it follows that man, whom He created in His image, is likewise a spirit (and eternal). It seems, then, that man later came into the earth as a physical being (Genesis 2:7): "Then the Lord God formed a man from the dust of the ground, and breathed into his nostrils the breath of life. Thus the man became a living creature."

The first creation for each of us is spirit. The next creation: a living creature formed from dust. It appears, then, according to the biblical story that we were inhabitants of the spiritual realm long before we entered the earth.

The Cayce material tells the same story, but adds the explanation—which really opened up my mind—of not one, but many entries into the earth, the idea of reincarnation. This idea is based upon the soul as an eternal being, having its origin in the spiritual realm and entering and leaving the earth plane over and over again, ostensibly to find its way back to a oneness with God, as Jesus was one with the Father. The background on this portion of the story also comes from the Bible: Jesus prayed for protection from the Father for His disciples, and "that they may be One, as we are One." (John 17:11)

With these three concepts as a foundation, I gradually built a view that incorporates the mind as a builder and choice as the ability to find our way through the earth experiences. The concept is better portrayed as a diagram or an illustration, shown on p. 90. It needs to be walked through point by point, for it shows not only the view of how things seem to work this lifetime, but the concept of time and how past incarnations with their experiences (similar to the present lifetime) are carried forward as memories and tendencies that influence each of us every day.

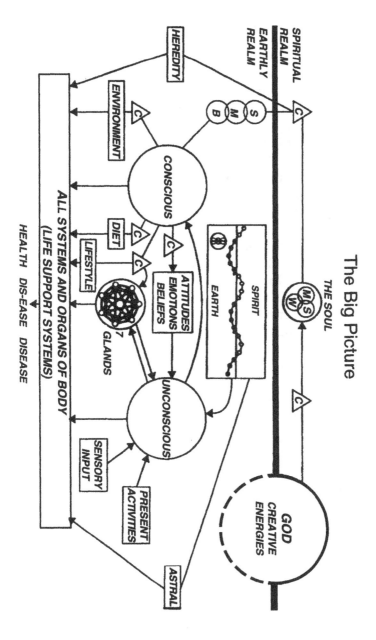

The Big Picture

The Soul's Journey Through the Earth

We have already indicated (in an earlier illustration, p. 3) that God chose to bring us as souls into being. The "S" represents the Spirit, the God-part that brings us life. The "M" represents the mind, the part of us that is always the builder. We can use it or abuse it. It is there, nevertheless, and it works always to build what we choose to build. The "W" is the will, or the greatest gift God has given us—the ability to choose. In this gift lies the power to move us to the condition Jesus called a Oneness with God.

Creation of us as souls came about in a dimension that some say is not limited by time. Difficult for me to understand, certainly. But this concept is sprinkled throughout the readings and also referred to by Jesus in John 14:26, when He promised that the Holy Spirit would teach us "everything," from the beginning. Did He mean the beginning of the earth—when it was formed?

Cayce, having read the Bible once for every year of his life, and drawing (in the course of his readings) from what he called the Universal Consciousness, gave his interpretation of that particular Bible verse. And it was meant for each of us, having eternal life. We were there before the world was formed and will be around when the earth has finished its plan in creation. This is what Cayce had to say:

. . . "He that takes my yoke upon him and learns of me, with *him* will I abide day by day, and all things will be brought to remembrance that I have given thee since the foundations of the world, for thou were with me in the beginning and thou may abide with me in that day when the earth will be rolled as the scroll; for the heavens and the earth will pass away, but my word shall *not* pass away." The promises in Him are sure—the way ye know! 262-28

In the illustration on page 89, most of the activities and choices below the horizontal line are understood to be found in this present incarnation. The same format happens every time we enter the earth. Other incarnations as part of our journey through time can best be shown as the travel of the soul (small circles, box) in and out of the earth, accompanied in the earth plane by the body (the "X" factor). We—our souls—are always in existence, even when we leave our physical bodies behind.

If we have been in existence since the beginning—before the earth was formed—we could say we are well over five billion years old in earth time. Time as it exists in the spiritual world, however, may be a different thing to comprehend.

Time doesn't seem to be important, however, because if we need to be here in order to learn how to be more loving, God's patience is sufficient to deal with our trials and our failures, no matter how long these may take. So we keep on meeting ourselves in lifetime after lifetime, through eons of time, building habits or patterns of activity—positive or negative—that keep us here until we learn the lesson of love as it permeates every fibre of our being and every moment of our life.

Each time we leave the spiritual realm, we become souls with bodies and we then go through the kind of choices seen in the illustration, using our mind as a builder and watching how our unconscious often dominates our responses in the earth. Why does this happen? Because we choose to let it happen, rather than choosing how we wish to respond. We react from the realms of our unconscious minds, according to the habits of attitudes, emotions, and beliefs that we chose to build into that part of our minds. In that manner, we tend to react habitually to most of the life situations that we encounter. This is shown in the arched arrow sent from the unconscious mind to the conscious.

But look in the illustration how the conscious mind can build with its choices. We first of all chose the parents we were born to—and that happened while we were still in the spiritual dimension. That's how we chose our heredity. We choose our diet consistently. And, in moving along the path to overcoming arthritis, we need to look carefully at the foods we consume. We choose, in a multitude of ways, what our lifestyle is at the moment and what it will become. We even choose our environment, internal as well as external. If we say, for instance, that "I didn't choose this horrible climate—my husband got transferred here and that's the problem." Well, who chose your husband? You took him for better or for worse. But always remember—you chose him. We choose our internal environment in a variety of ways. The food we eat, the kind of air we bring into our lungs. The sleep we get or don't get each night. Our exercise. The way we think. The way we react. We are indeed a very complex being.

In our daily activities we create habits by repetition. We choose to learn how to ride a bicycle or drive a car, or pitch a baseball or throw a batter out at first base—or whatever. These are things we want to do or like to do, and we choose to make them into habits in our unconscious mind—patterns that dominate and perfect themselves in the widespread nervous system of the body. We become expert at anything by repetition, feeding it into the habit/pattern area of our unconscious mind, over and over again. Very helpful in leading a productive life in so many, many ways, or perhaps giving ourselves unhealthful and disturbing repetitions and habits.

Our unconscious mind is very powerful in influencing our body and how it functions. It always has a direct effect as shown in the illustration. This comes about through the habits of movement that we have learned— driving a car, for instance, or protecting an aching back in lifting heavy objects by lifting in a certain way that becomes habitual.

The unconscious mind, in a sense, contains the awarenesses of the endocrine/glandular centers of the body, where the emotions dwell. These are shown in the center of the illustration and will be explored more extensively in the next chapter. We know that a danger alerts the adrenal gland instantly, and the body reacts almost entirely under the life-preservation mode created by the adrenals—totally changing the manner in which the internal functioning organs and systems respond. We fight or we take flight—or perhaps we find ourselves immobilized, frozen, and unable to respond. That is the learned response of the body built into the power of the adrenals. The action or inaction is the result of past choices which organize the adrenals to do the bidding of the overall mind with its learned responses. It may be fear, anger, defense, power, paralysis, depending on what has been taught the unconscious in times past.

The most important manner in which we use this power of choice, however, comes in choosing our attitudes toward situations and people; the emotional responses that we desire to manifest in appropriate times; and certainly our beliefs that guide our lives in so many ways. These learned responses—positioning themselves comfortably in these glandular centers—have a great deal to do with how the physiology of the body functions, and even more important, how we relate to people and situations in the outside world. This is always a major part of our Spiritual Journey, for we create either harmony or discord in the world around us and the same character of influence inside our bodies. Sooner or later our bodies respond with either health or dis-ease.

Also shown in the Soul's Journey through the earth is an astral influence, which might be described as influences of a mental nature coming from experiences and learning achieved between earth lives in the spiritual dimension.

Since the systems and organs of the body (shown in the illustration) are influenced by the heredity, the environment, the activities of the conscious mind, the diet, the lifestyle, the glandular/emotional content, the unconscious mind with all its patterns, as well as the astral influences—it becomes more understandable how each individual is truly unique and unequaled. The reactions, the responses, the physiological activities create in their own manner a completely different situation as far as health, dis-ease, or disease is concerned. The body certainly can restore health again, but it is not always simple.

Healing by Visualization

Nearly fifteen years ago, a woman moved to Phoenix. Three years earlier she had an operation to remove her right fallopian tube, which had been severely damaged from an infection. The same infection also involved her left fallopian tube to such an extent that it was closed from adhesions, making it no longer possible for her to become pregnant—according to her surgeon. The right ovary was later removed and she was told that there was also a small cyst on the remaining ovary. It was nine months later that she arrived and became a patient in the Clinic. She had been experiencing discomfort in the region of her left ovary. An examination revealed she had a large, lemon-sized cyst that was causing her trouble. She did not want to have surgery again.

Her therapy regimen consisted of visualization—seeing that cyst gone—and meditation, castor oil packs on the lower abdomen regularly three or four days a week, and a diet that aided the immune system by emphasizing the alkaline-reacting foods. (This is basically the kind of a diet that was discussed earlier in this book for arthritis.)

In three weeks her cyst had shrunk to the size of a Ping-Pong ball, and in two months it was gone. With these exciting results, she began to wonder whether perhaps the left fallopian tube might be following that same path of healing. She didn't particularly want to get pregnant, but with the assurance she had from her obstetrician that she could not possibly conceive, she stopped taking her birth control pills.

That was March 1984. In January 1985, she discovered she was pregnant! Several months later, her healthy eight-pound baby girl entered the world, excited, I'm sure, about *her* remarkable journey.

So this woman, using only her mind and two or three therapies designed to help her physical body, first cleared up an ovarian cyst, then liberated a fallopian tube from extensive adhesions. This, of course, allowed an ovum to course down its natural path, meet its mate, and bring into being a new channel for a living soul. Think of all those lymphocytes and macrophages that must have been swarming around the thick layer of adhesions, cleaning up debris, breaking down substances that were out of place, and rebuilding the normal anatomical structure of her errant fallopian tube.

This story, of course, has nothing directly to do with arthritis, but it does remind us that healing of the body has nothing to do with what has been diagnosed as cyst, pelvic infection, arthritis, or whatever—rather it demonstrates that the functioning of the body can be reversed so that it becomes constructive instead of destructive. And we call that healing.

Edgar Cayce said many times all healing is a divine event within the consciousness of the cells and the very atoms of the human body. We are on a return visit to the earth, finding an opportunity behind every illness to learn how to love. Isn't this really the way things happen? We experience a difficult disturbance of the physical body, but so often still have trouble accepting the rich dividend to be gained by living out this event and its healing process.

We may choose to be frustrated and perhaps bitter about having an illness, or we can accept it and through the course of events learn how to be gentle or forgiving or patient as we are healed. And sometimes we do not even know we are choosing grace instead of karma. Consider how excited and enthusiastic this young woman was when she experienced the disappearance of a cyst in her ovary! And then, despite her being told she could not conceive, she became pregnant and had a beautiful baby. She had karma, apparently, that in some way was dissipated, relieved.

The Cayce readings tell us *no* karmic debts from other sojourns or experiences enter in the present that may not be taken away in that, "Lord, have Thy ways with me. Use me as Thou seest fit that I may be one with Thee." (442-3) His ways are love, and that love is our ultimate destiny, so we must come to the manifestation of love sooner or later. Why not now?

Biofeedback and More Visualization

Biofeedback does not treat the body as many obviously think, but rather teaches the individual mind how to send messages to the body, which allow the conscious mind to change and bring about better conditions in the body through the voluntary control of involuntary forces. What is meant is simply that we are able, with training, to consciously control the speed of our heartbeat, for instance, or the temperature of the skin. It has been found that most areas of the body can be influenced consciously. One of our biofeedback specialists brought about a healing in his own body after suffering severe facial damage in a car accident. He used only the techniques he teaches his patients. The healing of the skin tissue amounted to a regeneration, so perfect was the skin afterward.

Dr. Elmer Green at the Menninger Foundation in Topeka, Kansas, pioneered much of the very early research in biofeedback. It was there that one of the most remarkable examples of healing by visualization came about. A boy who had an inoperable tumor of the brain was treated with radiation to the maximum allowable. The tumor increased in size in spite of the radiation. His parents were given a dismal prognosis of maybe several months to live. Using his mind, then, this lad literally visualized his tumor away under the careful direction of his therapist and friend, Patricia Norris, Ph.D. (*Why Me*, Stillpoint Publishing, Walpole, N.H., 1985) It took a year, but the young man is now free of his tumor.

How could this work by itself in arthritis? The joints and the structures affected by this malfunction of the physiology are as much a part of the body as the human brain and its attachments. With some individuals, I'm sure, the results would be excellent. In others, however, the results might be disappointing without some physical help from the diet, the exercise, and some of the other aids that might be used. It depends, of course, on what the patient might indeed believe about his or her own capabilities or, of course, whether the techniques being used are optimum.

As mentioned earlier, biofeedback does not treat the body but teaches the mind to control one of the body functions. Temperature control of a finger, for instance, can be monitored by attaching a thermistor to the finger. Then, as one concentrates, or relaxes, or moves the body, or relaxes the shoulders, or makes the mind calm, one can see the temperature of the finger going up or down on the thermistor. One continues working with the body until able to produce the desired effect.

The thermistor registers the temperature of the finger; that is, it gives feedback on what the subject's body is doing, and this is why the procedure, of course, is called biofeedback. Many body activities can be monitored and feedback given in the form of sounds or readings on an instrument, and thus one can learn what to do oneself to cause the body to perform this or that function. It may be by simply closing the eyes that one relaxes better; the biofeedback instrument would then give verification that one is attaining a relaxed state. Suggestion to the body may be given, such as, "My shoulders are warm, relaxed, and comfortable."

Heartbeat rate can be controlled in this manner; high blood pressure can be lowered; skin potential and temperature can be altered—even the activity of the lymphocytes in the bloodstream can be controlled by these methods. These are called autogenic exercises and can be developed almost as a habit or a thought form or a pattern in the unconscious mind, to be called on at will.

Guided imagery is closely related to visualization, perhaps is even the same thing. In group sessions, members of a group are led into experiences which are often highly meaningful.

It was in such a session once that I was able to contact my father, who had died eighteen years earlier. I saw him from behind, sitting at a drawing board, working. I called him, but he only seemed to hear something—a note or a voice, perhaps. But when I called him again, he was startled and stood up; he looked off in the distance where he saw a light. He picked up the hat he used to wear all the years before he died at age seventy-three and off he went, seeking the light. He looked younger, maybe aged forty or forty-five, than when I last saw him alive.

Dreams in the Healing Process

Your Spiritual Journey would not be complete without the recall, study, and application of the dreams you have every night—what they mean in your life and what their instructions might be concerning your physical body. We may not like what the dreams are saying, but the messages always seem to be valid and applicable in our lives.

We need to remember, also, the dream state occurs in a portion of the mind we ordinarily do not access, but this part of our beings is able to communicate with the consciousness of any other part of the body, as well as reach out to other minds and get in touch with the divine, which some call the superconscious mind. Dreams can look forward in time, as in precognition, as well as show us portions of our past lives that might aid us. Nearly all dreams are helpful in one way or another.

More than 600 Cayce readings were devoted to dream interpretation, and in one of these Cayce's sleeping mind was asked how *we* should interpret dreams. He answered, of course, that it depends to an extent upon the physical condition of the body. In other words, if one is ill and looking for help from within, then the dream state

will produce the help asked for. He added that we
should:

> Correlate those truths that are enacted in each
> and every dream that becomes a part... of the indi-
> vidual, and use such [for the purpose of] better de-
> veloping, ever remembering [that] develop means
> going toward the higher forces, or the Creator. 3744-
> 5

Dreams and visions are what we would call today very
close relatives. Cayce's perception was that dreams, visions, and the like are but activities in the unseen world
of the real self. We could say that "thinking" something
as one is in a semi-waking state is not just a "daydream"
but part and parcel of what the unconscious is wanting
to bring to our waking consciousness. Thus we expect
visions and dreams to have their origin perhaps in the
past, but maybe in the present, or even portraying what
the future holds for us. Since we are whole entities—
body, mind, and soul—then we need to recognize that
dreams involve us at every level of our being. Yet to the
unconscious mind there is no past or future—only the
present, and all that exists can be drawn upon and used.
    Cayce reminds us, too, we are able to see from a differ-
ent perspective—through the dreams and visions—the
experiences we find entering our lives. And it seems this
man constantly brings us back to essentials:

> [Through dreams] the entity may gain the more
> perfect understanding of the relations between God
> and man, and of the way in which He, God, mani-
> fests Himself through mankind. 900-143

In the biblical story of Jacob's son Joseph, whose travels eventually took him from Canaan to Egypt, he is probably best remembered for his dreams, some of which angered his brothers. He was sold to the Ishmaelites for twenty pieces of silver by Midianites who had rescued him from the pit where his brothers had thrown him. Joseph ended up in Egypt as a servant to Potiphar, a captain of the Pharaoh's guard. After being falsely accused by Potiphar's wife, Joseph spent time in the dungeon of the Round Tower. His interpretation of the Pharaoh's servants' dreams led him two years later to the Pharaoh, who had a puzzling dream no one could interpret. Joseph told him the dream predicted seven plentiful years were coming, and then seven years of famine. This led to Joseph becoming governor of Egypt. It's a tremendous story that cannot be told in a few words, but one that shaped much of the history of the Old Testament. You can read it in Genesis (chapters 37 through 50).

Dreams have proved invaluable to inventors, and always to those who pray for help in times of crisis. There are precognitive dreams, which tell of the future, and there are dreams of past incarnations which can be helpful in many ways to the dreamer.

There are dreams of guidance and dreams of what might be happening to cause illness in the body. In the ancient world, kings and emperors sought for guidance through their dreams. In recent years research has shown that everyone dreams every night, and needs only to prepare the sleeping mind to bring the memory back to waking awareness in order to utilize the power the dreamer created within his or her own being.

A friend of mine dreamt he went into the basement of his house, thinking something was wrong. He found the drain pipes from the toilets were all stopped up. In asking him what might be bothering him physically, he told me he had been constipated for a long time.

Another patient was plagued for months with a severely disabling bursitis in both shoulders. He had been to a series of doctors to no avail. His search for healing led him to reading about reincarnation and karma, and he found that often karma surfaces in the present as physical difficulties. One night he had a dream (he thought it might really have been a vision because of its content) in which he asked: "Is this condition karmic in origin?" A voice answered: "No! Lift up your arms!" At that point he awakened and found both his arms lifted high over his head, a position he had been unable to assume consciously for months. He has had no bursitis since.

A close friend of mine told me about a recurrent dream that was more like a real experience. The first time he experienced it, however, was during a meditation. He found himself walking down a misty path, hearing gentle music while he moved along. He didn't know where he was going, but he knew it was all right. When the mist cleared he found himself in front of a beautiful chapel. He thought it should be a cathedral, but it was too small. He walked inside and there in front of him stood the figure of Jesus, who beckoned to him to enter and to take a seat in front of a semicircle of seated persons whose faces or identity he could not make out. Then he was face to face with Jesus, and they had a deep conversation. He couldn't recall what was said, but he knew it was important, for his life was different from that point on.

How do we deal with experiences such as that? What do they mean? If you were to have such an encounter, and you were working with your physical body and its difficulty with arthritis, how would you interpret it?

Might it not mean your soul was living through an experience telling you that you really are an eternal being, participating in this earth plane in a physical body? And you would be encouraged to continue the work you are doing, for as Jesus said, with God all things are possible. The emotions would certainly be healed in such an experience—since emotions are part of the glandular structures of the body and directly influence the workings of the body's physiology.

6

What About Your Attitudes and Emotions—Where Do They Fit In?

↩

How can one's attitude create an illness in one's body? An attitude could be defined as a stance taken toward any aspect of the life we are presently involved in—a stance built out of repetitive choices made in the near or the far distant past. We could also call an attitude a point of view taken on one of life's situations.

It may be an attitude born out of the teachings we were given as children. A child is told, for instance, never to trust strangers. The parents, of course, are instructing the child in what they think is best without recognizing they might be leading their loved one into a habit of distrusting everyone, not just strangers. This attitude gives the child the opportunity to experience fear, which was probably brought forward from past lives in his consciousness so it could be met. In one sense, it is constructive. But it is clear that the attitude of distrusting strangers and the emotion of fear are interlocked.

These influences are difficult to understand, because we are not used to thinking of emotions and attitudes as being carried over from one lifetime to another. We are not used to thinking of these qualities as lodged in the cells and in the consciousness of the endocrine glands of the body. Nevertheless, they are. And they have a direct effect on the physiology of the body, which in turn can manifest abnormalities and create illness. Cayce talked about it in simple terms. As the child we have been talking about grows up, the emotions of fear and hate—its partners certainly—might breed specific illnesses, as in this reading:

> To be sure, attitudes oft influence the physical conditions of the body. No one can hate his neighbor and not have stomach or liver trouble. No one can be jealous and allow the anger of same and not have upset digestion or heart disorder. 4021-1

The body is generally built through the attitudes that have been habitually made a part of the unconscious mind, so that we deal with life and with the physiology of our bodies in such a way that the illness we "get" is designed particularly for us from the way we have thought and felt and reacted to our environment. In the case of arthritis we have frequently kept our fears and angers inside, buried deep in the unconscious mind, suppressed and essentially forgotten. But they don't go away—they remain inside. What happens then is our bowels, under the control of our unconscious mind and its autonomic nervous system, keep their contents likewise inside the body and unconsciously slow down or hinder the eliminations. As we have already indicated, lack of proper eliminations brings about the condition we call arthritis.

The portion of our unconscious mind (our emotions, attitudes, and belief patterns) that brings about these physiological changes is lodged in the endocrine glands. Thus, what we think, feel, and experience—all this stuff our senses relate to us—becomes directly and, in a major fashion, related to our physiology and thus to our health or lack of it.

Cayce spoke to this aspect of our true nature when he reminded us it is always the response, the reaction that is sought when we are trying to better ourselves. It is in those reactions to life's situations that we are able to see what we have programmed into our unconscious mind and what direction we have chosen to take in past incarnations and in the present.

Our attitude toward certain foods, for instance, shows how we can unknowingly hurt ourselves. If we were brought up to think of meat and potatoes as the staple of our diet, then that's what we feel we "should" eat, and we like it. Our response to salads might be negative but by eating salads as a regular part of our diet, we might overcome a major portion of our tendency toward arthritis. Such a change would help bring the body into a better balance physiologically.

Attitudes are extremely important in any phase of life. When I was a medical student on the OB rotation, I was caring for a woman who had delivered her baby less than twenty-four hours earlier. She kept saying she was going to die. She seemed depressed, but fearful of dying. My chief resident scoffed at what the woman was saying, pointing out to me that all her lab findings and blood pressure were normal. The next morning she was dead, and I'm not sure the pathologist really found the cause of her death. This woman knew something, of course, that we cannot yet fit into the scientific mode. But she knew it.

About ten years ago a hot controversy was touched off in medical circles by Barrie Cassileth's study published in the *New England Journal of Medicine* and an accompanying editorial by Dr. Marcia Angell. Both stated that patient outlook plays no role in the course of cancer or the survival of the patient.

The editorial (312:1570-1572) held that any relationship between disease and the mental state or attitude is largely folklore. National publications picked up the story and amplified its meaning. Then the other side of the story began to appear as researchers and individuals rose to the defense.

A British study by a team at Kings College, London, showed that, in fact, attitude may be the most significant single factor in survival of breast cancer patients. Many in the field of psychoneuroimmunology responded, citing the multitude of studies done in that field which give evidence that thought and emotion affect the immune system. I'm sure every thinking physician today recognizes that the patient's attitude influences the course of every disease.

Attitudes are of prime importance in the Cayce readings. Attitudes speak of hope and faith, of joy and belief, of understanding and forgiveness—of many things. They also lead us to destructive activities if they are loaded with qualities such as anger, jealousy, fear, revenge, and the like. Attitudes are products of the mind that relate human beings to their source or move them in the opposite direction. Very powerful, the need is always there to pay attention to attitudes one has chosen to hold close in his interpersonal relationships. Cayce's readings consistently remind us to view the other person—*any* other

person—with the awareness that he or she, like us, was also created by the Universal Forces, in God's image.
Cayce gave a reading for a man who apparently had a long-standing lung disease. The physical recommendations were offered first and then Cayce added his psychological dissertation:

> To be sure, there should be rather that expectant attitude of the body; not to become overanxious at the slowness and at those detrimental conditions that continue to be in the attitude of the body as related to general conditions. But begin to *plan* as to what the body will *do* when and *as* the improvements come; for unless there is the expectancy, unless there is hope that is given, first the spirit and then the body—and then the activity in the mind of an individual life and its manifestation and its outlook becomes a drag, a drug on the hands of one that is being attacked from within, as we would say, by the dis-eases of a physical body. But hope and trust and faith in the Divine within, that may find manifestations in all the applications that may be made for the revivifying, the rejuvenating of that spirit of life and truth within every atom of the body, will put to flight all of those things that hinder a body from giving expression of the most hopeful, the most beautiful. Not only be good; be good *for something!* Hold to that which is of Truth! 572-5

In other words, Cayce was simply advising this individual to do the things the physical body needs to be cared for, but first things first. Let your attitudes be corrected and follow what Jesus said nearly two thousand years ago: "Seek ye first the kingdom of God . . . " (Matt. 6:33) All the other things will be added in due time.

After suggestions were made in reference to the man's pathology, Cayce ended his reading with the instructions once again that spoke to his higher self and his direction in life—these could not be separated from his physical self:

> ... follow the outlines as indicated here, not leaving off those that are helpful—but follow these, knowing and seeing—not as rote in doing this or that at any particular time, but knowing—that the spirit of truth, of God, is manifested in the life flow not only of self but of those things that would create in the atoms of the body itself the awareness of His presence being and abiding with thee. So, unless these be builded with a mind of service to Him ... who is the Giver of all good and perfect gifts, who maketh and taketh away Life itself. *Put* thyself, thy life, thy troubles, in His hand, and have Him—*through* those influences of His life upon the life of individuals in the world—*mould* thee into a life of service for Him. 572-5

To touch another person is very often a physical manifestation of a desire to be of aid or comfort. A hug is like that. A Johns Hopkins School of Medicine study, reported by William E. Whitehead and his associates, maintained that being physically touched will not only make you feel better, it will also lower your heart rate, let it just loaf along doing the job more easily of supplying blood to the rest of the body. Just placing a hand on someone's wrist is likely to lower the pulse rate, whether at home or in the doctor's office. They observed also that if you touch a person who is in pain, the physical contact minimizes the extent to which the pain drives up the heart rate, even though it does not lessen the pain. So it may be that a hug a day indeed keeps the doctor away. Or at least bring more ease to the body.

The Body's Hierarchy of Function

Who's in charge of our body, anyway? To whom should we go when we need to have something "fixed" in this ailing body of ours? My professors in medical school had no problem with that question. "Go to your doctor, of course." He has more knowledge than most and should be best equipped to help. Since I was to become a physician, too, I had no difficulty with that approach, because I learned thousands of facts, ideas, syndromes, symptoms, and specialized names to be used when we got into practice. That seemed reasonable.

Yet the question of getting the body "fixed" seemed paramount, and we medical students were taught about many drugs, many procedures—but there was no specialty called "Therapy." Different parts of the body were given specialty ratings, like the neurologist, the gynecologist, the orthopedist, and a number of other experts in body parts. There was also the internist, whom we understood as the diagnostician. This specialist was highly regarded by the general practitioner; being like a detective in a murder mystery. But I still found no specialty in medicine called "Therapy."

I accepted the things which were taught me for the most part, yet I kept thinking, "Isn't therapy what people come to the doctor for? To be helped?" All we had in the '40s were drugs, radiation, and surgery, with some hangover herbs and procedures from the early days. We did not think about attitudes and life experiences as causing physical problems. And we did not ascribe to the endocrine glands the capacity to have consciousness and to take part in the healing process. Or to cause disease!

That's the picture I was given five decades ago in looking at the world of healing around us, and it has continued for many, many years. Not much has changed, really, except for the improvement in techniques and diagnosis given by the scientific world. Medicine has a way of negating the spirit—not recognizing the human as a spiritual being traveling in a strange land. And, in the halls of medicine, the emotions and their direct relationship to the physiology of the body is considered to be, for the most part, imagination on the part of the patient, or perhaps a problem to be left at the doorstep of the psychologist. But what I was taught had nothing in it to explain what a human being really is.

We are souls created in the image of God and living many lifetimes in these three-dimensional physical bodies often as strangers, sometimes not knowing ourselves, but most certainly as voyagers through time and space on a journey to discover the truth and to recognize our destiny. And illness is always a part of the journey.

This awareness gives us a whole different perspective from which to view arthritis. There is something beyond this physical that we cannot see with our eyes or feel with our hands, relate to with our voice and our ears. It's that which created us as body, mind, and spirit and beckons us to find the divinity that exists in every atom of our body cells. This kind of thinking helps us to understand why arthritis can be seen as a Spiritual Journey.

We desperately need, in these years ahead, to look within—rather than somewhere outside—for the power that moves our bodies. Those who would counsel us to look elsewhere are leading us astray, no matter how many academic degrees they may have, or how much knowledge they have accumulated.

We have already established that Cayce offered us as fact the idea that every organ, every cell, even every atom has consciousness, and each seeks to do its part in this complicated and wonderful unit we call the human body. Logic will say, then, that among all these different functions being performed within these bodies of ours, someone has to be in charge. This is where the hierarchy of the body comes into play. We need to know more about our bodies, where choices can be made, where influences have their origin and their effect. But first of all, how is hierarchy defined? The *American Heritage Dictionary* gives four choices, depending, I'm sure, on the situation. Definition of a hierarchy:

1) A body of persons organized or classified according to rank or authority.

2) A body of entities arranged in a graded series.

3) A body of clergy organized into successive ranks or grades with each level subordinate to the one above.

4) Ecclesiastical rule by a hierarchy.

Since each tiny bit of tissue in our bodies has a degree of consciousness, with knowledge of how to do the job it's been assigned to do, I think we could consider organs or systems to be persons in the first definition and then see if there might be reason as to how the body is functioning physiologically.

Most people might rank the mind or the brain as highest in authority. From what we have covered in this book thus far, this might seem true, for we speak of the mind as the builder, and we most often think of the brain as housing the mind. (Not totally true, of course, for the mind reaches further than just the brain, but that's the most common concept.) In the Cayce viewpoint, mind exists in every part of the body. The mind is very important and should be placed near the top of the hierarchy.

In looking at the body's physiology, however, I've chosen to place the seven endocrine glands (as a unit) at the apex of the hierarchy. For they have more power and more direct influence on the rest of the body's functioning than any other system or any single organ including the brain.

The conscious mind, as the overall director of the body, is shown in the second illustration (p. 89) as using the power of choice to create in the unconscious mind the attitudes, emotions, and beliefs the individual wishes to create—as mentioned earlier—through repetitive use of those qualities in one's life in relationship with other people and situations.

However, the unconscious mind, or at least the emotional part of the unconscious that dwells in the endocrine glands, has more direct effect on the physiology than does the conscious. At times the conscious mind can, with a certain amount of difficulty, override the involuntary activities, but reactions, responses, reflexes come about without the conscious mind taking part. Our conscious mind, by choice, creates the kind of responses the body makes, certainly, but the glands and their indwelling emotions and feelings dominate when the physiology is concerned. And it is done without us knowing at a conscious level, most often, that this is happening.

In the illustration included in chapter 5, you'll see these glands are located very much in the center of things. They are shown to be part of the unconscious mind and are impacted by the conscious mind. They are shown as a unit to influence the life support systems, for better or for worse. There are, of course, seven other factors which affect the physiology. As might be noted, all of these other influences as shown in the illustration (with the exception of the astral) were chosen by the mind at one point or another, utilizing the power of choice.

You came into the earth; you chose your parents.

That's your heredity. Your environment—also chosen—always affects your health to one degree or another. Dietary influences are obvious. Your lifestyle—the way you've patterned your life—alcohol, smoking, and stress—have their importance and affect the body. Both your conscious mind and your unconscious can move you this way or that. But let's deal with the seven glandular centers of emotion, attitudes, and beliefs.

To understand better how they get involved with the life support functions of the individual who has arthritis, we might consider how they might work together, recognizing that they all have a consciousness of a sort. It may be like seven members of a family relating to one another. No individual of such a unit relates to others in the same manner. So it is with the glands. They create, in a sense, a family, all having their say in what happens in a given experience in the world outside, or where any physiological function of the body is involved. An attitude of cooperation or coordination, for instance, established through the seven members, would tend to move the body functions toward a state of health and harmony. The dissention, the dissenting attitudes, on the other hand, would bring a disruption and eventual disease or illness.

In much the same manner, the habits of emotional response, attitudes, or belief patterns always govern how we treat our fellow humans, how we create in our environment a feeling of harmony or discord. In other words, we unconsciously create that which builds or that which destroys in the world around us—unless we *choose consciously* to apply the emotion, attitude, or belief we know within ourselves is the best we can offer. When we do choose, we must agree to be satisfied with the result, no matter what it may be.

The seven glands, then, act as a communicator between the outside world and what is happening inside as the life force works to keep us healthy if we will let it. And they become participants in both worlds, inner and outer. How can we ever believe that feelings of any sort do not influence either our health or the people and environment which surrounds us all the time?

We are *always* changing. Thus we are always becoming healthier or on the path toward illness. No matter what the physical problem may be that has surfaced, the overall picture demonstrates the mind can choose to create a new, more positive package of attitudes in the unconscious in the process of dealing with relationships. And the seven glands are the domain of the attitudes, the emotions, and the beliefs.

Change can then start a movement of the forces within the body toward becoming healthier. Or we could say we become closer to our normal state of good health. For good health is what we were given in the beginning of our Earth experience.

The glands, then, manifesting the attitudes, reign supreme over the body physiology, given that they always work with the tools—or the patterns of the attitudes and emotions—that have been given them. These glands react to what they *are*. The conscious mind *acts* through choices.

How would we visualize or gain an idea of what happens in the interior of an endocrine gland when it acts or when it is being patterned and is developing a new approach to life? Some call this pattern a thought form. It gains strength as it is repeated. All habits do this. But in the substance of the energy pattern which the Cayce information calls a spiritual center or a glandular center (known better in the East as a chakra), there appears to be a flow of divine energy coming into the gland to be distributed throughout the body through the nervous

system and, at the same time, through the hormones released into the cardiovascular system

The entry into the gland appears to some who see
such energy patterns as a vortex. Each of the seven
glands is associated with a vortex. Then an interesting
thing happens. The energy entering the body through
such a system is pure, unadulterated, divine in its nature, part of our relationship to God for we are a manifestation of God. In the gland, however, there are these
thought forms, the attitudes and emotions in energy
form. Some of them are in tune with the divine energy—
some are not, and these are in need of change. For, as
they exist in the present, they create a disturbance and a
muddying of the divine energy, so the messages given to
the body through the nervous system and the bloodstream are confused, giving improper information. This
is the manner in which illness has its beginning.

Each of the glands, of course, sends out hormones
through the blood. We know, too, that each of the endocrine organs is a neurohormonal transducer, linking the
nervous system and the vascular/hormonal system together in action. Thus each gland sends information
through neurological impulses to every cell in the body,
while supplying those same cells with hormonal, biochemical influences, undoubtedly the most powerful
chemicals supplied to the body for its use.

Perceived in this manner, it becomes understandable
that the glandular centers occupy a critical position of
influence as the life force—called the Spirit in the Cayce
material—is distributed in consciousness to the entire
body.

In one sense, then, the glands deal with the life of every individual, while the mind shapes by its choices what
the life will be, both inside the body and in the world
outside. So, what comes first, the life or the mind? From

the perspective the Cayce readings offer us, the hierarchy of the body places the Life Force at the top, with the mind using that life to create what is desired.

The Immune System and Its Role in Arthritis

Several years ago, after speaking at a college of alternative healing in Minnesota, I was being driven back to the airport. We passed over a small stream of water I would have called a creek back in Ohio, my home. I glanced at the sign just before we crossed the bridge—it read: "Mississippi River."

"What does that mean?" I asked my host. I knew what the mighty Mississippi River is like—I lived alongside the Ohio, and that river is magnificent by itself, but not near the grandeur of the river that divides the East from the West in this country. But this creek?

"Sure," he said, "it's the Mississippi. It starts just ten miles north of here." I was flabbergasted! The following year, I made it a point to see where this mighty river originates, bubbling out of the earth and creating a wee stream. As a matter of fact, I walked across it, just so I could tell the story. There were maybe six or seven rocks I stepped on so I could cross the river without even getting my feet wet. Quite an experience!

The lymphatic stream in the human body—an integral part of the immune system—is much like the Mississippi or the Ohio. It has its beginning in the outer reaches of the body where cells live together and do their work. The cells take in food and oxygen from the arterial capillaries (smallest vessels in the arterial system) and give off their products into the intercellular spaces. These cellular yields are partly substances that are helpful to the body, and some are products of metabolism, better known as wastes. The capillaries cannot receive most of the cellular harvest because of their molecular size, so they end up being part of the lymphatic stream.

In the case of Mississippi, water comes out of the ground to start the river. In the body, lymphatic fluid comes out of the cells, and the lymphatic stream begins. It takes lymph from places all over the body, and becomes known, after passing the cisterna chyli in the abdomen, as the thoracic duct, ascending through the diaphragm into the thorax to empty into the left subclavian vein. The lymph then becomes part of the venous system which eventually, after moving through the heart and lungs and becoming the arterial system, delivers its good things and its waste products in the proper places as it moves through the body. It picks up oxygen in the lungs, giving off carbon dioxide and other minute substances as we breathe.

Thus we can understand that the arterial system of the blood gives life to the cells, and the lymphatic and venous streams take away the end products of the ongoing activity in the cells.

The thymus, one of the endocrine glands, is the director—the boss—of the immune system and is located in front of and slightly above the heart in the mediastinum. Lymph glands throughout the body are part of the system; they are located for the most part in line with the flow of the lymph, acting as cleansers of the lymph in some areas. Other lymph nodes create white cells which are also part of this far-flung system. The liver, spleen, tonsils, adenoids, appendix, and Peyer's patches are understood to be important parts of this system.

What does the immune system do? What is its purpose? Simply put, the immune system is a protector of the body, preventing alien cells, bacteria, etc., from attacking the body. The lymphocytes—when the immune system is healthy—kill cancer cells that happen to be in the tissues of the body. It is those same lymphocytes that help rebuild the body.

The immune system, then, protects, rebuilds, and generally keeps the body healthy. Quite a task. We need to remember, as pointed out earlier in this book, the lymphatic stream functions at a pH level higher than the bloodstream. So it is our responsibility to maintain that level, so the body might be more easily kept healthy. Exercise, diet, attitudes, and a host of simple therapies, if chosen wisely, can and often will enhance the immune system, which is just beginning to be recognized in the scientific community as the key to both maintaining and regaining a state of health in the body. Scientists searching for the answer to AIDS have stated publicly that we have been looking in the wrong direction. What is needed is to turn our attention to the immune system, not to the HIV virus.

It is undoubtedly best to realize that the God Force which flows through each of us has the power of producing health in any condition of the human body, *if* we do not obstruct its flow. That's a big *if.* It implies we need to learn to adopt a lifestyle that recognizes what we are here for in the first place, and that we must learn to love both God and our fellow humans. This has much to do with the immune system, one's personal state of health as well as the impact it has upon the world in general.

It is not surprising that two-thirds of the Cayce readings deal with troubles in the human body. For the body, the mind, and the spirit or soul has a destiny to be One with God, and every activity is meaningful in that direction.

In the Edgar Cayce material, the human is seen as a spiritual entity, a unique combination of body-mind-spirit manifesting in this material world. The nature of the evolved human being—one who is moving closer to his or her spiritual destiny—is truly manifested by the

manner in which we treat our fellow beings. How much
kindness, gentleness, love, understanding, and forgiveness is one using day in and day out? In the case of the
evolved entity, the answer is "Much, indeed." These
qualities are loaded with constructive emotions, and the
one whose life encompasses these regularly has discovered the way to a healthy body.

Qualities such as those just listed are part of the plan
to keep the immune system at the proper pH level, for
the thymus has been called the heart center and is the
part most affected by sensitive, feeling kind of events
such as losing a loved one, being rejected, etc. We need
comfort, we need to be accepted, we need to be loved,
and we need to give love, acceptance, and comfort to
others. This is the way the thymus center maintains its
health and its proper acid/alkaline balance.

Any major accident, any surgery, any experience
which is traumatic touches the consciousness of the individual at the level of the thymus. Because of the
trauma and the fear involved, the experience creates turmoil in all the glands and elicits a response, either helping out in the healing of the body through the positive
attitudes that have been gradually taught to the emotional centers or creating blocks to healing. Any one of a
multitude of therapies might be offered toward healing,
but none can heal if the individual rejects it as an aid.
That's how powerful we each are in this world of our own
we have created.

Atomidine and Its Uses in Arthritis

The early Edgar Cayce readings provided information
for the formulation of a substance known as Atomidine.
It is an iodine preparation, but there were other substances added which improved the activity of the

Atomidine in balancing the body functions and was said to be less toxic than any other form of iodine. It was suggested as a benefit for the body in a variety of ailments over the course of the nearly half a century of Cayce's career in giving readings.

Among the conditions Cayce mentioned are: anemia, arthritis, poor assimilation, asthenia, asthma, baldness, blood building, boils, bursitis, cancer, tendency to cancer, canker sores, cataracts, circulatory problems, cysts, general debilitation, dermatitis, eliminatory problems, diverticulitis, goiter, hay fever, hirsutism, malaria, prostatitis, plus many others.

Iodine, it seems, is a vital element in the makeup of the human body. Medical research confirms this opinion, but does not cover many of the uses that Cayce saw as appropriate, nor some of the ways in which iodine benefits functioning at the cellular level of the human body. The readings state that iodine is essential to the process of building new cells (cell division). Reading 636-1, which discusses baldness and the restoration of color to the hair, tells what goes on inside the body when Atomidine is taken:

> The Atomidine—that is activative in the glands, especially the thyroid, the adrenal and all the ductless activities through the atomic forces in iodine, the one basic force with potash—makes for a balance throughout the functionings of the body itself. 636-1

Balance in the endocrine glands is essential to the health of the human body—this we know. So, if we take Atomidine, the readings say these glands will at least be in better harmony than before the iodine was taken.

It is interesting to read how changes occur within the

body. For example, for a case classified simply as "Acidity," Cayce recommended:

> ... one drop of Atomidine in half a glass of water before the morning meal, and the next day three drops of Glyco-Thymoline in water before retiring ... Alternate these ... and within a few weeks the acidity of the system will be changed, and also the vibrations through the glandular forces that control the lymph circulation in alimentary canal as well as organs of the pelvis ... the Atomidine acts as a gland purifier—causing especially the thyroids and the glands in the stomach, particularly the pyloric portion of the stomach and throughout the duodenum, to change in the form of secretions thrown off—and this affects directly the circulation. 3104-1

Some years ago I suggested a treatment for a sixty-nine-year-old man who had such a stiff neck that in order to look around he had to twist his entire shoulder girdle. His neck would not allow for flexion or extension, nor any movement laterally in either direction. Immobilized by cervical spinal arthritis for some years, he wanted relief. My suggestion was to change his diet a bit; start doing the head-and-neck exercise twice a day; and to start using Atomidine.

Faithful in following directions, he experienced a gradual improvement—and within two years he could flex and extend his neck with the best of the younger people. And his neck was not limited in rotation. He took one drop of Atomidine in half a glass of water Monday, two drops Tuesday, three on Wednesday, four on Thursday, and five on Friday. He rested from medication on weekends and resumed the same routine Monday for three weeks each month.

At the A.R.E. Clinic, we adopted the above regimen after studying some seventy-five different methods of taking Atomidine mentioned in the readings. It was difficult to determine what was best for each individual, but this particular therapeutic program has brought positive results in many cases.

In the instance of a sixty-one-year-old woman who had developed arthritis, Edgar Cayce told her to have massages and manipulations, Atomidine, hot Epsom salts baths, and alcohol and peanut and olive oil rubdowns. Her manner of taking the Atomidine was "one minim [drop] of Atomidine in half a glass of water before the morning meal, and the same upon retiring . . . " (1512-1) She was told to increase the dosage to two drops the following day; three on the third day, four on the fourth day, and five on day number five, morning and evening in each case. After taking the Atomidine, she was to take a hot Epsom salts bath, using ten to twenty pounds of salts, and immersing the entire body. After the bath came a vigorous rubdown, then a massage with a mixture of oils and then alcohol. This five-day routine was followed by a five-day rest before repeating the routine twice more.

Before turning to Edgar Cayce for one of his readings, this Alabama woman had been to New York specialists and to Hot Springs, Ark., but "gradually grew worse," her nurse reported. After trying Cayce's recommendations "she is now walking without a cane," according to the nurse. "She really is very much better."

When healing follows the use of Cayce's unorthodox approach, it is always a fascinating experience. In cases where the endocrine glands need balancing, Atomidine seems to be one of the real assets in the pursuit of good health. Without balance and coordination in the glands themselves, peace and harmony throughout the body cannot be a part of the picture—and healing comes only with difficulty.

Meditation in the Healing of the Body

In our Temple Beautiful Program, we always have meditation as a group after early morning exercises. It prepares the day for us and, after meditation, our breakfast becomes more of a meaningful event as we bless our food and then discuss our dreams of the previous night. This following quote from the readings gives us much to think about especially concerning meditation and the way we really are:

Enter ye in at the gate called straight, through thine own preparation in thine own manner, and meet Him there. For thy body is the temple of the living God, of thy living soul; thy body is the temple that must be, should be, *will* be kept holy, if ye will know thy true relationships to thy Maker.

Keep the trust thou hast in the *All*-Creative Forces; knowing He is able to keep that thou committest unto Him against any experience that may arise in thine own activity.

Keep the self in such a manner as to be circumspect in thine own consciousness. Be true to self, making for those activities that bear the fruits of the Spirit; just being kind, just being gentle, just being patient, just showing fellowship, just showing brotherly love; just bearing witness in thy walks, thy acts, thy understandings unto thy fellow man. And ye shall know Him face to face. For He hath promised to bring to such the *remembrances* from the foundations of the earth, of the world, of the universe. For thou wert in the beginning, even as He. 261-15

When we meditate, there is a movement of energy from the lowest of the endocrine/spiritual centers up alongside the spine toward the head. It is felt that this energy meets an energy that comes in from above at the level of the pineal gland, creating light and what is called the mystical marriage. The pineal is also called the third eye; it is sensitive to the light from the sun and creates difficulty for us when we travel by plane and experience jet lag. Meditation is attuning the physical and mental bodies to their spiritual source. To help me in visualizing what happens in meditation, I see my energy rising along the spine and attuning itself to the creative energy of God that is always flowing through me. When we allow our physical bodies to become quiet and let our minds cease their endless meanderings, we are in the state where attunement can take place. Sometimes in your meditations you may feel as if the Divine has actually given you a new understanding. This has happened so much that some teachers say meditation is listening to God and prayer is talking to God.

However we may understand the practice of meditation, we can readily accept the idea that meditation brings us closer to the Divine, closer to understanding the nature of the Divine, and thus further along the path of our journey in understanding our own nature. If indeed we are created in the image of God, then our inherent nature, our soul nature, is like God and has powers yet undreamed of. We can awaken our conscious mind to what we truly are and begin to manifest it in our lives. Meditation is the act of bringing those energies and vibrations that make up our being into closer communication and attunement with God.

The Edgar Cayce readings were once termed "Ten Million Words from an Unconscious Mind." That was the title of the first lecture I heard (in 1955) about the mate-

rial which became the foundation of my work in the field
of medicine.

Those who have been working with this material in
Virginia Beach at the A.R.E. Library compiled portions
of the readings under various titles, and the Library Series of twenty-four books gradually became available.
Two of these volumes contain readings dealing with
prayer and meditation. If you are interested in finding
out what Cayce said about this subject, you will need to
direct your search toward volumes two and three of this
series, which contain nearly two hundred thousand
words. This is obviously a large and important area of
exploration.

In relating prayer and meditation to the endocrine
glands of the body and to attitudes and emotions, we
need to see ourselves as individuals who are manifesting the Spirit of life itself, the Life Force, and doing it with
knowledge or without knowledge of the nature of God,
nor of ourselves. Meditation is a means of direct communication with the Source of Life, and thus it becomes
a necessary part of our Journey—whether we deal with
life as a whole or simply the meanings behind and correction of a physical condition such as arthritis.

I want to include in this portion of the book a very
short reading about meditation or prayer; and another
that stimulates your imagination, perhaps, or your desire to know more. First, Cayce once told a thirty-eight-
year-old man that "Meditation is listening to the Divine
within." (1861-19)

Then, to the group working with the readings at the
time the study groups had already begun, Cayce offered
them instruction in this manner:

To each of you , then, we would give a word:
Ye all find yourselves confused at times respect-

ing from whence ye came and whither ye goeth. Ye find yourselves with bodies, with minds—not all beautiful, not all clean, not all pure in thine own sight or in thy neighbor's. And there are many who care more for the outward appearance than that which prompts the heart in its activity or in its seeking.

But, ye ask, what has this to do with Meditation? What *is* Meditation?

It is not musing, not daydreaming; but as ye find your bodies made up of the physical, mental and spiritual, it is the attuning of the mental body and the physical body to its spiritual source.

Many say that ye have no consciousness of having a soul—yet the very fact that ye hope, that ye have a desire for better things, the very fact that ye are able to be sorry or glad, indicates an activity of the mind that takes hold upon something that is not temporal in its nature—something that passeth not away with the last breath that is drawn but that takes hold upon the very sources of its beginning—the *soul*—that which was made in the image of thy Maker—not thy body, no—not thy mind, but thy *soul* was in the image of thy Creator.

Then, it is the attuning of thy physical and mental attributes seeking to know the relationships to the Maker. *That* is true meditation. 281-41

Cayce went on to ask, in a rhetorical manner, how would you, as an individual "go about learning to meditate?" He talked about the fact that there must be parts of the physical body acting as contacts with the soul self or the superconscious mind that is part of God. These contacts are the centers we have been working with in this chapter and they are essential to our Journey in Consciousness. And we go about learning to meditate by simply sitting down at a quiet time, closing our eyes, letting our bodies and our minds become quiet, and attuning. This is how we start.

7

Let's Put It All Together

⤳

We can indeed go on a Spiritual Journey and find in the process a healing of the arthritis which may have afflicted us for a period of many years. The manner—the how—in which this might come about is the subject of this book. But let's always remember, the process of overcoming arthritis is first and foremost a journey of the Spirit. For you are called on to remember that you—the soul that is you—have been in the earth through many incarnations, seeking, seeking, always seeking for something that has seemed to elude your questioning mind.

Strange, indeed, it would be if the answer to your inquiry were found hiding behind those aching bones. They might be giving you a wake-up call. Maybe we simply need to be more loving!

In considering arthritis as a Spiritual Journey, we might listen as Cayce describes healing—all healing—in this way:

> For, all healing comes from the one source. And whether there is the application of foods, exercise, medicine, or even the knife—it is to bring [to] the consciousness of the forces within the body that aid in reproducing themselves—the awareness of creative or God forces. 2696-1

It has been vitally important for me to probe into the unconscious images Cayce presented about what we are as human beings. I felt I *had* to understand the body functionings better. The "forces" of elimination, for instance. All tissues, you see, are composed of atoms, and it was Cayce's point of view that all atoms have consciousness. Consciousness is a force when applied in any situation. Thus Cayce looked at those consciousnesses that were moving these aggregations of atoms and cells and he called them "forces." And they, knowing their origin after being awakened by the Divine in a healing experience, respond by attaining their normal status—that which they really had in the beginning. Some people call this a healing or a cure.

Healing can be thought of as a combination of the cleansing of the body functions, a greater purifying of the mind and an attuning of the body and mind to the Creative Forces of the Universe. Interesting, isn't it, that it doesn't just amount to taking a few pain pills or having an adjustment or a massage or receiving the laying on of hands in prayer or going through a visualization experience. It's an encounter in the ongoing stream of life, which Cayce likened to a pool that may refresh and replenish one this time around.

What About the Healing of the Body, Then?

How shall we look at this wonderful creation with its need to be healed? Certainly we can see it as a body-mind-spirit entity—and as a oneness that encompasses all of these. But more than this, shouldn't we look at the body as an ongoing stream of consciousness, a creation constantly changing even as we think about it? The body needs to be seen as a process of attuning itself to its true nature, helping it to aim itself toward the destiny of being a companion with the Father-God.

Do these, as we have indicated . . . Not as rote, but knowing that within self must be found that which may be awakened to the *building* of that necessary for the body, mentally and physically and spiritually, to carry *its* part in this experience. For the application of any influence must have that which is of the divine awakening of the activative forces in every atom, every cell of a living body. 726-1

True healing is not a simple thing. We can bring healing to any part of our bodies, but unless we reach deeper, into the very nature of the patterns, the consciousness, that activates the physiology of the body into creating the problem and then *start* reversing the process, we have not really begun. As we manifest in our lives those fruits of the Spirit that the readings frequently talk about, true healing comes about. For we *are* on a spiritual journey.

Karma and Its Part in Healing

We have really been on this kind of a journey throughout the ages, appearing over and over again in the earth, with new mothers and fathers, sisters and brothers. But we always are instinctively moving in one direction: toward oneness with the Universal Forces that we call God.

In the process we have misfired, in a sense, in trying to do things which today we would call good or constructive. In trying to understand our children, for instance, we may not have recognized them and acknowledged them as being created in God's image. They did something "wrong" and we had to punish them! Or we let anger get the better of us when we were trying to understand why our spouse strayed from the straight and narrow in another relationship.

Many thoughts come to mind when we consider the way we should act toward another person and we failed to do so. Kindness or gentleness were simply forgotten— the forgiveness which is so important in all of our lives.

Today we say, "What goes around, comes around." Or what we sow, we also reap; or that we are experiencing the law of cause and effect. Many ways of recognizing the law of karma. We can expect our attitudes and emotions that have been activated toward others at some point in time (maybe way back in another incarnation) to return to us today in our daily activities and experiences with other people. We haven't really lost much, however, for we have been forgiven by a God who loves us and thus are offered another chance. The mishaps, whether we recognize them or not, come back to roost on our doorstep. It's called karma, and we must always meet it in our relationships, no matter where or when this might occur. However, Cayce suggested all karma could be met in an easier, more beneficial way:

Karmic influences must ever be met, but He has prepared a way that He takes them upon Himself, and as ye trust in Him He shows thee the way to meet the hindrances or conditions that would disturb thee in any phase of thine experience. For, karmic forces are: What is meted must be met. If they are met in Him that is the Maker, the Creator of all that exists in manifestation, as He has promised, then not in *blind* faith is it met—but by the deeds and the thoughts and the acts of the body, that through Him the conditions may be met day by day. Thus has He bought every soul that would trust in Him. For, since the foundations of the world He has paved the ways, here and there entering into the experience of man's existence that He may know every temptation that might beset man in all of his ways. Then in that as the Christ He came into the earth, fulfilling then that which makes Him that channel, that we making ourselves a channel through Him may—with the boldness of the Son—approach the Throne of mercy and grace and pardon, and know that all that has been done is washed away in that *He* has suffered that *we* have meted to our brother in the change that is wrought in our lives, through the manner we act toward him . . .

No karmic debts from other sojourns or experiences enter in the present that may not be taken away in that, "Lord, have Thy ways with me. Use me as Thou seest fit that I may be one with Thee." 442-3

So we ask, "What are God's ways?" Peace, harmony, joy, understanding, gentleness, forgiveness. But then, you can look at them as fruits of the Spirit, and better yet, experience them in your life. For they are the manner in which these misdeeds of the past can be set at rest.

Let's Review a Bit

Balance needs to be restored in the body if we wish to ask it to function in a "normal" manner and be healthy. The need exists to bring healing to the bones, cartilages, and ligaments and ease the pain, but the physical treatments require the aid of our mind and our emotional reactions to be successful. We must develop in our unconscious minds (and in the glands) the reactions that will not only help at the present time, but will build gradually the kind of responses to life's interpersonal relationships that will create for us forward movement in our soul's journey toward oneness with God.

We need to learn to look at life as an opportunity to grow, to become more loving, to use each experience as an opportunity for soul growth. We can learn and appreciate the fact that we are eternal beings, having our origin in the spiritual realm in the image of God, and entering the earth plane time and again to learn how to be more godlike.

We need to learn that our destiny is to know ourselves to be ourselves yet one with the Creative Forces or God. In other words, we can begin to understand that we are here in the earth as visitors, making our way moment by moment through the experiences that we encounter, finding what it was inside ourselves that led us to have this kind of an experience which we call arthritis.

We can learn to accept ourselves as we are, being content in where we are in consciousness, but not satisfied. We can use the arthritis we have developed—or any illness for that matter—as a time for inner searching, learning how to love our fellow humans and God. Simple, isn't it?

What About the Eleven Steps?

1. The arthritis diet. This diet stimulates the liver as part of its action on the physiology of the body. It keeps the body tissues slightly on the alkaline side, which accentuates the ability of the immune system to rebuild and to protect the body. The rebuilding is always a necessity—otherwise, the arthritic lesions could not be regenerated.

With all the wonderful happenings taking place inside the human body, we know the diet forms the very foundation of what is required to overcome the condition we call arthritis.

2. Epsom salts baths. This is the second step in influencing the body using physical applications. The skin is one of the four eliminatory organs and is actually the largest of all four. The other three are the kidney and urinary tract, the liver and the intestinal tract, and the lungs and the rest of the respiratory system. With the hot Epsom salts baths, the respiration is speeded up, the skin perspires heavily, the circulation to the liver and kidneys is speeded up as the body heat increases the pulse rate and the activity of the heart. All are good reasons, certainly, to use this therapy.

3. Exercise! Don't forget the body always needs some activity in the way of exercise. Again, circulation of blood and oxygen throughout the body is a benefit to the rebuilding of the tissues, when done in a reasonable manner.

4. Use castor oil packs on the abdomen. Although the packs may only be used an hour a day, three days consecutively each week, don't underestimate its value. Anything that enhances the immune system activity must be looked at as valuable. The degree of value may vary with individuals, but it is always there.

5. Iodine is an essential element in the body. Remember, the Cayce readings imply that a better balance of function among the seven endocrine centers in the human body is brought about by Atomidine. And keep in mind that these same glands are part of our emotional nature and have much to do with hormonal and neurological function in the physiology of the body.

6. Dreams can be of much greater value if they are recalled, written down, and made the subject of interpretation. Cayce said that anything important that is going to happen in our lives is foretold in the dream life. We can discover significant past-life experiences in our dream life. Make it a habit to pay attention to your dreams.

7. Visualization and biofeedback techniques aid the mind in taking an active part in the healing process, as well as giving us an insight into our own unconscious minds.

8. Work with attitudes and emotions. This is the third aid in healing arthritis that involves working with the mind. The emotions give us insights to be gained, whether they are positive or negative aspects of the unconscious mind that either need to be let go of or enhanced. We build our personality through the use of our mind and our will, and our health and our degree of soul growth depend to a great extent on what we choose to put into our unconscious mind as patterns or thought forms.

9. Healing by touch. Everyone who desires to help another person be healed has some degree of healing in their hands, whether it be the masseuse or the osteopath, the chiropractor or simply the hug you may give or receive.

10. Prayer and meditation is an essential component of the journey toward healing. We need to remember

who we are, where we originally came from, and what our destiny is. Recalling that makes for a closer attunement with the Divine, which leads us to develop a more health-producing lifestyle.

11. Consider joining a study group that will help each individual to apply concepts of soul growth and healing in daily life. People working together can help each other bring about a more balanced lifestyle, a greater awareness of their inner selves and, through meditation and prayer, they can find their lives enhanced in many ways. (The A.R.E. sponsors a study group program worldwide called "A Search for God," complete with books and study aids. Information can be obtained by calling the Association for Research and Enlightenment in Virginia Beach and asking for the Study Group Department.)

One More Thing

I would be remiss in my suggestions for healing arthritis if I did not acknowledge the mass of information available to the public at the present time on arthritis and on healing in general. There are many approaches to healing in this country, without looking at other cultures and countries and their developments to bring comfort and health to their peoples.

I've been closely associated with other medical doctors, of course, including osteopaths, chiropractors, acupuncturists, naturopaths, physical therapists, masseurs and masseuses, spiritual healers, prayer groups, music therapists—just to mention a few. *Alternative Healing* (Kastner and Burroughs, Halcyon Press, 1993) identifies more than 165 approaches to the practice of the healing arts. It seems more are discovered or invented every day. So an approach to healing arthritis is not uncommon.

However, an approach that puts together a concept of

our origin as a spiritual being spending repeated incarnations here on the Earth and seeking to find our true destiny while searching for meaning in an illness such as arthritis—this, I believe, is a unique approach. I used this quote earlier in the book, but it bears repeating:

> . . . all healing of every nature is the changing of the vibrations from within—the attuning of the Divine within the living tissue of a body to Creative Energies. This alone is healing. Whether it is accomplished by the use of drugs, the knife or whatnot, it is the attuning of the atomic structure of the living cellular force to its spiritual heritage. 1967-1

Every human being is creative; and you may find Cayce's kind of attunement in simply one or two of the steps I outlined for you. There are a multitude of other therapies that may be helpful. But whatever therapy program you might eventually adopt, please always remember that you are on a Journey offering high rewards—not only at the end, but during the process of awakening those cells to their spiritual heritage.

What's to Be Learned from Arthritis?

In offering us insights into how our material body gets involved with something as common as arthritis, Cayce reported on the suffering and torment that arise from a war inside our own bodies. His description is unique in that he reminds us there is the spiritual part of ourselves that continues to seek for the ultimate, while the physical part wants its way in this material world. And these two parts create havoc through the war they are engaged in:

In the physical we find that of the material manifested conditions, and those conditions that worry
and prevent happiness are produced often by the
mental and spiritual outlook; for, as has so oft been
given, the spirit is continually at war with the flesh.
Will one satisfy only the desires of the flesh, then
the mental and spiritual *must* suffer, and bring into
being—through that suffering—those conditions
that become as torment to the individual; for remember that it was said, truly, "though He were the
Son, yet learned He obedience through the things
which He suffered," and when an individual so attunes the mental, the spiritual life, as *not* to be in
accord with that element within self that demands
as much recognition as the purely material body,
then one must know that there must be the price
paid in that of discontent, of disruption, where faith
becomes shaken, where there comes the falling of
the idol of the eye, the shattering of hope, and that
intenseness often reaches such conditions as to
produce for the body that of sleeplessness, inability
to control emotions, inability to control even circumstances and self's own will—that gift of the
gods that makes mankind that as he is, that he may
be either one with or away from His presence. In
Him is peace, in His counsel is there faith, in His
light and in the shelter of His wing is there to be
found aid—mentally, physically, spiritually; for He
is faithful who has given "Will ye be my people, I
will be *your* God." 5469-1

Much can be learned in the process of overcoming arthritis. We can be patient with ourselves and with others.
We can search out who it is in our lives that has been a
real problem for us, remembering that we are always

meeting ourselves, and the enemy is not "them." One of
the readings I quoted told us that "what is meted must
be met."

Another interesting comment from this source of information was that everyone we meet is like a puppet in
our lives. Also, each individual becomes as a mirror for
us to look at and see ourselves. The puppet and the mirror are simply other ways by which we are being guided
to see ourselves. For we are indeed more different than
we think. We are complicated beings, but we are certainly interesting and deserve the best we can muster as
we heal our infirmities. It is best if we don't try to avoid
the reaches of that law of the universe which, when followed, leads us toward our destiny. This Cayce comment
seems to sum it up in a significant manner:

> Know, as you analyze yourself, these are unalter-
> able truths: God is, and to Him first you owe all alle-
> giance. Or you work with or against that Divine
> within. Not that ye separate God and become as a
> servant, but as the Master so oft indicated "I and the
> Father are one, I am thy brother, ye are cocreators
> with God. Be ye holy, even as your Father in heaven
> is holy." 5104-2

So, how is it that we are healed? What is the magic for-
mula? Do we need to look at our past-life experiences to
gain insight into the cause? Is that a requirement? Perhaps the answer is much more simple than we might
think. Possibly the acknowledgment of what we really
are is the very first step. We were created in the image of
God. God is love, and as we manifest love (as best we can)
in our relationships with others we meet day by day, we
are one with love, thus one with God. And healing
comes.

Appendix

‿

Castor Oil Packs

Materials Needed:
1. Wool flannel cloth
2. Plastic sheet, medium thickness
3. Electric heating pad
4. Bath towel
5. Two large safety pins

Instructions for Use:
Prepare first a soft flannel cloth (cotton flannel is all right if wool flannel is not available) that is two to four thicknesses and measures about ten-by-twelve inches after it is folded. This is the size needed for abdominal application. Other areas may need a different sized pack. Place the flannel on the plastic sheet which should be

slightly larger in all four directions than the flannel. Then pour some castor oil onto the cloth. Make sure the cloth is wet but not drippy with oil. Next, apply the cloth to the area that needs treatment, making sure the cloth is next to the skin and the plastic is on top, preventing the oil from soiling clothing or bedclothes.

On top of the plastic, place a heating pad and turn it on to low to begin with, then to medium or high if the body tolerates it. Then wrap a bath towel, folded lengthwise, around the entire area and fasten it with safety pins. (Best to do this while the patient is lying down.) The heating pad should remain in place between one hour and one and a half hours. The pack itself can be worn all night without the heating pad. Be extremely careful to avoid excessive heat! The idea is to help, not hurt.

The skin can be cleansed afterward by using soda water (to a quart of water, add two teaspoons baking soda). Keep the flannel pack in a plastic container for future use. It is possible to use the same pack for different problems, and it need not be discarded after one application, but check with your physician about specifics. It is best, after seven or eight uses, that the pack be washed.

Washing Instructions

1. Soak the pack in a solution of baking soda and hot water, using four ounces of soda to two quarts of water.

2. After the pack has soaked for at least 20 minutes, wring it out thoroughly. Then wash it separately in a washing machine.

Helpful Suggestions from the Edgar Cayce Readings

[Remember] There is as much of God in the

physical as there is in the spiritual or mental, for it should be one! 69-5

... when there is the tendency towards an alkaline system there is less effect of cold and congestion. 270-33

Do not have large quantities of any fruits, vegetables, meats, that are not grown in or come to the area where the body is at the time it partakes of such foods. This will be found to be a good rule to be followed by all. This prepares the system to acclimate itself to any given territory. 3542-1

... cereals that carry the heart of the grain; vegetables of the leafy kind; fruits and nuts ... The almond carries more phosphorus *and* iron in a combination easily assimilated than any other nut. 1131-2

Do not use bacon or fats in cooking the vegetables ... 303-11

Do have plenty of vegetables [grown] above the ground; at least three of these to one below the ground. Have at least one leafy vegetable to every one of the pod vegetables taken. 2602-1

Corn and tomatoes are excellent. More of the [vitamins] are obtained in tomatoes [vine ripened] than in any other *one* growing vegetable! 900-386

... Olive Oil in small quantities ... is a food for the intestinal system ... 543-26

. . . do not eat great quantities of starch with the proteins or meats. 416-9

Avoid too much of the heavy meats not well cooked . . . The meats taken would be preferably fish, fowl and lamb; others *not* so often. Breakfast bacon, crisp, may be taken occasionally. 1710-4

Q. How much water should the body drink daily?
A. Six to eight tumblers or glasses full. 1131-2

Bolting food or swallowing it by the use of liquids produces more colds than *any one* activity of a diet! Even milk or water should be *chewed* two to three times before taken into the stomach . . . 808-3

Well, then, each morning upon first arising, to take a half to three-quarters of a glass of *warm* water . . . this will clarify the system of poisons. 311-4

The cooking of condiments, even salt, *destroys* much of the vitamins of foods. 906-1

Certain characters of food cooked in aluminum are bad for *any* system . . . Cook rather in granite, or better still in Patapar paper [vegetable parchment paper]. 1196-7

Q. Consider also the steam pressure for cooking foods quickly. Would it be recommended and does it destroy any of the precious vitamins of the vegetables and fruits?
A. Rather preserves than destroys. 462-14

. . . *never,* under strain, when very tired, very excited, very mad, should the body take foods in the system . . . And never take any food that the body finds is not agreeing with same . . . 137-30

. . . what we think and what we eat combined together—*make* what we *are;* physically and mentally. 288-38

The Acid-Alkaline Balance

Alkaline-Forming Foods
All fruits, fresh and dried, except prunes, plums, and cranberries.

Apricots	Limes	Berries
Oranges	Dates	Peaches
Figs, (unsulphured)	Pears	Grapefruit
Pineapples	Lemons	Raisins

All vegetables, fresh and dehydrated, except legumes (dried peas, beans, and lentils) and rhubarb.

Asparagus	Olives (ripe)	Beets
Onions	Carob	Oyster Plant
Carrots	Celery	Rutabagas
Eggplant	Spinach	Green beans
Sprouts	Kohlrabi	Sweet potatoes
Lettuce	Tomato juice	Mushrooms
Milk, all forms	Cottage cheese	Cheese
Honey		

Acid-Forming Foods

Vegetable oils	Prunes	Plums
Cranberries	Rhubarb	

All cereal grains and their products
All high-starch and high-protein foods

Filberts almonds	Almond butter	Nuts

Legumes   Dried beans   Dried peas
Lentils   Meats   Lamb
Poultry   Chicken   Turkey
Guinea hen   Duck   Goose
Wild game   Visceral meats   Heart
Brains   Kidney   Liver
Sweetbreads   Thymus   Egg whites
                                  (yolks are not
                                  acid-forming)

References and Suggested Reading

A Search for God. Virginia Beach, Va.: Edgar Cayce Foundation, 1987.

Jesus the Pattern. Virginia Beach, Va.: Edgar Cayce Foundation, 1980.

McGarey, William A. *Edgar Cayce Remedies.* New York, N.Y.: Bantam Books, 1983.

Physician's Reference Notebook. Virginia Beach, Va.: Edgar Cayce Foundation, 1968.

McGarey, William A. *The Oil That Heals.* A.R.E. Press, Virginia Beach, Va., 1994.

McGarey, William A. *In Search of Healing.* Perigee Books, Berkley Publishing Group, New York City, 1996.

Oulette, R. *Holistic Healing.* Fall River, Mass.: Aero Press Publishers, 1980.

Rusznyk, Istvan, et al. Lymphatics and Lymph Circulation: *Physiology and Pathology,* edited by L. Youlten. 2nd English edition. Elmsford, N.Y.: Pergamon Press, 1967.

Kastner, Mark, and Burroughs, Hugh. *Alternative Healing.* Halcyon Publishing, LaMesa, Calif.

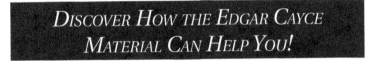